JOHN SHUFELDT

MD, JD, MBA, FACEP

LEADERSHIP
YOU

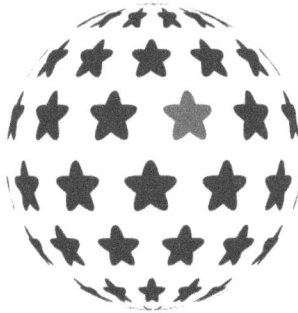

YOUR FUTURE STARTS WITH YOU

PUBLISHED BY OUTLIERS PUBLISHING

Inquiries should be addressed to:
Outliers Publishing
Hangar 1
7332 E. Butherus Drive
Scottsdale, AZ 85260

ISBN: 978-1-940288-72-7 Soft Bound

      978-1-940288-84-0 Hard Bound

      978-1-940288-73-4 eBook

Printed in the United States of America

Design and Composition: Perfect Bound Marketing + Press

Editor: Bob Kelly of Wordcrafters, Inc.

Chief Copyeditor: Kaleigh Shufeldt

Team Copyeditors: Maribeth Sublette, Amanda Best

Developmental Editors: Craig Kasnoff, Maribeth Sublette, Amanda Best, Amy White

Productions Editor: Amanda Best

Quantity sales, textbook and course adoption use:

www.johnshufeldt.com/contact/

Individual sales: www.johnshufeldt.com/leadership-bookstore/

For Michael and Kaleigh –

Thank you for being my continual inspiration!

TABLE OF CONTENTS

INTRODUCTION

"The one thing that you have that nobody else has is you. Your voice, your mind, your story, your vision. So write and draw and build and play and dance and live as only you can."

~ Neil Gaiman

British-born Neil Gaiman is a popular novelist and screenwriter, who has won numerous awards for his work. In the words I quoted above, he reminds us of our uniqueness and encourages us to take charge of our lives.

This adage has taken many forms: Be the author of your own book—the hero of your own play. Only you have the power to chart your own course or alter your own stars. The proverbs go on and on. The take-home point is this: Start now. The first step is often the most difficult, but once you start moving, that momentum takes over and things start happening and then they start accelerating!

Gaiman offers sound advice. Whatever goal, whatever destination you want to reach in your life, you have to lead the way. It's called self-leadership, and that's what this book is all about.

Think of this as Newton's first law as applied to mankind, "An object at rest stays at rest and an object in motion stays in motion with the same speed and in the same direction unless acted upon by an unbalanced force." Objects tend to "keep on doing what they're doing." In fact, it is the natural tendency of objects to resist changes in their state of motion. This tendency to resist changes in their state of motion is described as inertia. Self-leadership is the unbalanced force applied to help overcome inertia.

Now I'm not talking about being a lone wolf, a one-man band, or a lone ranger. On your journey through life, there'll be many others who'll help point the way—parents, teachers, friends, colleagues, teammates, mentors, and others. But, ultimately, you're the one to decide which road to take, hill to climb, pitfall to avoid, and challenge to tackle and to overcome. Remember, it's rarely the obstacle that impedes your growth, it's how you respond to that obstacle that determines your future.

That's what self-leadership is all about—the ability to influence yourself, overcome your inertia, and make changes for your own benefit and, ideally, for the benefit of others.

Before your journey begins, the conversation you must have with yourself is simply: "Here's where I see myself, and here's where others see me as well. And this is where I want to go." It may be a small change or it may be a huge one, with multiple steps along the way, and with multiple points on the path. But, there has to be the desire to want to align your stars, or rescript your future, or change your perspective to something else that you see as better for yourself and, hopefully, better for others as well.

Self-leadership can, in many respects, be more difficult than leading others, in the sense that the ability to change your habits, thinking, way of life, goals, and aspirations, is much more challenging than trying to convince other people to change theirs. Unless you can influence yourself, unless you can lead yourself to be better—and better can mean better at school, better at sports, a better person, more engaged, more empathetic, whatever it is you're trying to achieve— then it's unlikely you'll become the leader you were meant to be. Self-leadership has to come from within.

Trying to change others is a different matter, offering its own challenges. You've probably heard that old saying: "You can lead a horse to water but you can't make him drink." Well, that may be true, but, as someone has pointed out, you can always make that horse thirsty by putting some salt in his oats. In becoming a strong self-leader, the qualities you display can make those around you thirsty enough to want to follow your example. But they have to be the ones to initiate and continue to pursue the new behavior.

Self-leadership is within everyone's grasp. The late Bob Moawad, a world-renowned motivational speaker and author, once said: "The best day of your life is the one in which you decide your life is your own. No apologies or excuses. No one to lean on, rely on, or blame. The gift is yours—it's an amazing journey—and you alone are responsible for the quality of it. This is the day your life really begins." I will never forget the day that switch flipped for me. It was more than 36 years ago and I never looked back, other than to be grateful I recognized it when it happened.

Those to whom the concept of self-leadership comes easily are those who can will themselves into changes of behavior because, despite its difficulty, they see the long-term benefits. So, part of the skill is the ability to see a little bit over the horizon, where you can imagine yourself in a different place than where you are now. It's the ability to envision the future, putting yourself there, and saying, "This is what I want my future to look like." Ultimately, that future begins with you. You're the architect, the pilot, the owner, and the occupant. It's a great opportunity; don't let it go to waste.

In a magazine article I read recently, one highlighted comment caught my attention. Here's what it said: "We were lucky enough to grow up in an environment where there was always much encouragement … to pursue intellectual interests, to investigate whatever aroused curiosity."

Those words certainly describe the environment we live in today, but they were actually spoken about a century ago by a man named Orville Wright. Wright, with his older brother Wilbur, ignored the doubts and ridicule heaped on them in their quest to prove man could indeed fly. And fly they did, a feat that literally changed and shrank the world forever.

What kept them going? Wilbur answered that question this way: "We knew that men had by common consent adopted human flight as the standard of impossibility." But that word—impossibility—wasn't in their vocabulary, so the Wright brothers, a couple of determined self-leaders, broke through that standard and kept right on going.

Orville and Wilbur Wright were what one might have called "tinkerers" back in those early days of the 20th century. It's not a term we see in this Age of Technology, but to tinker means to "work with something in an unskilled or experimental manner." To me, it describes one who is "incurably curious." The Wright Brothers were curious men, who believed man could fly. They started tinkering with bicycles, then moved on to gliders, experimenting with a variety of wing shapes and sizes, and eventually launched their first gasoline-powered plane, the Wright Flyer I, made of spruce and covered in muslin.

As that first flimsy little plane left the ground on December 17, 1903, could they have possibly imagined that giant multimillion dollar aircraft, carrying hundreds of passengers all over the world, would one day dot our skies? Or that giant rockets would carry men to the moon—and beyond? Perhaps not, but they were willing to take those first steps—to lead the way, whether anyone would ever follow them, or not!

What is it you're incurably curious about? What "standard of impossibility" might be in your path as you face the future? What would you like to do to change the world? The opportunities have never been greater than they are today—right now! You can—literally—hold the entire history and wisdom of the world in the palm of your hand. There'll never be a better time to get started than right now. So, what are you waiting for? Take that first step to becoming the leader you're meant to be.

I often include the following quote in my talks on self-leadership: "Someone once told me the definition of hell: The last day you have on earth, the person you have become will meet the person you could have become." And this quote by Friedrich Nietzsche is in the footer of every email I send out: "The individual has always had to struggle to keep from being overwhelmed by the tribe. If you try it, you will be lonely often, and sometimes frightened. But no price is too high to pay for the privilege of owning yourself."

In the pages that follow, we'll describe many of the qualities of the self-leader, and share with you the stories of some individuals whose lives model those qualities—men and women of all ages, who dared to tinker, to explore, to dream, and to discover. We hope their stories will excite and encourage you. As Orville Wright said, "to pursue intellectual interests, to investigate whatever arouses curiosity." Remember: Your future begins with you!

CHAPTER 1

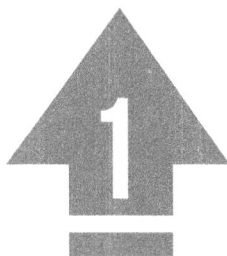

HUMILITY: THE ELUSIVE VIRTUE

*Humility stands alone among the virtues in that
as soon as you think you have it, you don't.*

~ John Dickson

I'm going to let you in on a little secret I've learned repeatedly over the past 35 years—those who have to scream their accomplishments to others are generally the most insecure. Allowing your own sense of self-worth to rest solely upon your achievements and the accolades of others is a sure way to ultimately be uncertain, anxious, and fearful.

Now here's another little secret you probably already know: nobody likes a bragger. Or elitists. Or just plain arrogant jerks. I've known plenty from all camps, and try as I may, I've never understood their rationale. I'm not saying I associate only with the Mother Teresas of the world. My friends have chosen to spend their time with me and, as a result, are subjected to my version of humor, which I'd venture to guess Mother Teresa would not have appreciated. Nonetheless, my friends are great individuals who don't feel the need to convince everyone around them of their greatness by constantly boasting of their deeds, successes, or awards.

1

I like to surround myself with humble people, and not just because I loathe gloating. Humble people care about others. To get a sense of a person, I sometimes ask in an interview, "Which type of person are you? Do you run toward a threat or away from it?" Maybe the answer, at least partially, describes one facet of humility. I want the people I work with to care not only about the task at hand, but also about other people. When a team is made up of individuals who choose to forgo their own status, and preconceived notions of others, incredible progress can be made, while having a lot of fun.

So why is humility important? It actually empowers you. By foregoing a prideful heart, you allow yourself to take risks. Moreover, people trust and respect humble people and finally, humility allows you to open yourself up to learning something from everyone and everything.

When I think about the most influential and successful people I've encountered, nearly all of them are genuinely humble. It seems to me that genuine greatness goes hand in glove with humility, a trait that on the surface seems like it would quiet the desire or ability to achieve distinction. One must never make that mistake, though. Humility is not a sign of weakness. It also certainly doesn't indicate a lack of desire or ability to achieve amazing things. In fact, I'd argue that humble people might even have an edge when it comes to achieving success.

I challenge you to think about the type of person who comes to mind when you think of the virtue of humility. Is this a trait you hope to embody? I hope so. It's something I strive for daily. I also challenge you to think about your concept of confidence. The best self-leaders can embody both traits with class and ease.

When you really think about it, confidence is needed in order to embody humility. Confident people are self-assured. They have faith in their own abilities. They don't need acclaim or constant reassurance from others in order to feel whole. Thus, there's no need for them to boast or brag. Humility and confidence naturally go together. They're like the peanut butter and chocolate combo of virtues. They might not seem like a natural pairing, but once you've put them together, it's obvious they were meant for each other.

THE HUMILITY CONUNDRUM

In the Introduction to his book, *Humilitas, A Lost Key to Life, Love and Leadership*, from which the opening quote was taken, Australian teacher and author John Dickson notes the difficulty in identifying those who are truly humble. He immediately follows those words by adding: "And, yet, the reverse does not follow. *Not* thinking yourself humble is no indication that you are. You might be right! Both the arrogant and the humble are unlikely to think of themselves as humble. So how could you ever know if you have attained the virtue?"

I think we could all agree that humility, elusive as it is, can never be self-conferred, nor can it be achieved in solitude. Dickson defines it as: "the noble choice to forgo your status, deploy your resources or use your influence for the good of others before yourself."

This is key. Humility doesn't mean bowing to others or living your life in servitude. It simply means you don't spend your life promoting or boasting about yourself.

Humility is not thinking less of yourself,
it is thinking of yourself less.

~ C.S. Lewis

Humility is an important quality for the self-leader to develop, for several reasons. First of all, it's freeing. Humility makes you secure in the knowledge that you're on a level playing field with everyone else.

Second, it makes you fearless. If your ego is removed from the equation, then trying new things, exploring, failing and trying again becomes a game, as opposed to something to be feared.

Third, humility helps build teamwork. When team members recognize that everyone shares both the credit and the blame, they step up their game and hold one another accountable.

There are several ways self-leaders demonstrate their humility. They never take sole credit for whatever is accomplished. Instead, they share the credit with everyone involved. They never talk about themselves, but are quick to brag about the members of the team, and they lead by example.

Humility means two things. One, a capacity for self-criticism...The second feature is allowing others to shine, affirming others, empowering and enabling others.

~ Cornel West

Just prior to defining humility, Dickson writes: "It's worth noting the way it pops up in some unexpected places." Based on stories I've heard or read, these places would include such widely separated locations as a jewelry store in Australia, and high on the slopes of the world's tallest mountain, involving two famous men who saw no need to impress others with their achievements.

 In *Humilitas*, Dickson tells a story about multi-billionaire Bill Gates helping an employee in a jewelry store in Australia figure out how to reboot the store's sales register. As he worked on it, she said to him, "So you know a little bit about computers, do you?" Instead of mentioning his pioneering role as co-founder of Microsoft, he simply nodded and completed the transaction.

AN "AVERAGE" BLOKE

The other story is about famed mountain climber Sir Edmund Hillary of New Zealand. With his Sherpa guide and friend, Tenzing Norgay, Hillary became the first to reach the summit of Mount Everest, the tallest mountain on earth. On a later climb, while posing for photos on the mountain with several climbers, Hillary had another climber stop and inform him that he was holding his ice axe incorrectly. So he allowed the man to adjust the axe in his hand, thanked him and continued on with the picture-taking. Onlookers were amazed.

Sir Hillary got it right. When I think about this story, I'm even more impressed by his response to the unaware, know-it-all observer. What positive would come from Hillary letting that man know of his accomplishments? Surely, the man would've been greatly embarrassed, but would Hillary be adding anything positive to the exchange? He had the confidence in his own abilities, achievements, and therefore, had no reason to publicly shame the know-it-all.

Yet, such modesty wouldn't have surprised those who knew him. Standing atop Mount Everest, which 15 earlier expeditions had failed to reach, and where many experienced climbers had lost their lives, Hillary had recorded the momentous occasion *not* by having his picture taken, but by taking one of Norgay. When asked why he didn't have his guide take one of him, Hillary explained: "As far as I knew, he had never taken a photograph before, and the summit of Everest was hardly the place to show him how."

Their feat brought both men instant worldwide fame. Newly crowned Queen Elizabeth II of Great Britain promptly knighted the 33-year-old Hillary. However, Sir Hillary was not about to rest on his laurels. He continued the mountain climbing he loved and took part in an expedition to the South Pole. He played an active role in environmental and humanitarian causes, many of them on behalf of the Nepalese people, working tirelessly to raise funds for health and education projects in their country.

Hillary remained very much in the public eye for more than a half-century after Everest, and was regularly described in world media as "a hero," "a living legend," and "the world's greatest living explorer." But he'd have none of it. "I have never regarded myself as a hero," he often insisted, "but Tenzing was."

On November 5, 1998, at a dinner hosted by the American Himalayan Foundation in San Francisco, he told the audience: "I was just an enthusiastic mountaineer of modest abilities who was willing to work quite hard and had the necessary imagination and determination. I was just an average bloke; it was the media that transformed me into a heroic figure. And try as I did, there was no way to destroy my heroic image. But as I learned through the years, as long as you didn't believe all that rubbish about yourself, you wouldn't come to much harm."

Trust yourself. Create the kind of self that you will be happy to live with all your life. Make the most of yourself by fanning the tiny, inner sparks of possibility into flames of achievement.

~ Golda Meir

FLYING WITH BATMAN

So there I was (all great aviation adventures start out this way) flying through an intense thunderstorm on my way back from a meeting at Drake University. I'd only had the jet for a few months and was required by insurance to have a "check pilot" along for the ride. The young woman who was my usual check pilot had a conflict, so retired America West Airlines Captain Larry Newman took her place.

All the seats were filled. The radar showed moderate to severe thunderstorms directly along our path and the XM weather showed the cloud tops at 50,000 feet, about 9,000 feet higher than we could fly. In short, we were in for a wild ride. I turned to the passengers and made a motion of waves with my hands. They all understood and cinched their belts tighter. I was nervous but fully engaged at the tasks at hand. Larry was impassive.

I didn't know Larry. He didn't talk or share much. Given what little I knew of his past, he was clearly competent—anyone flying as a captain for a major carrier is rock solid. For the next 30 minutes (or what felt like two hours), we were tossed around like a cork in the midst of a wine-dark sea on a stormy night. Larry never touched the controls and when I had a question, he simply said, "It will be fine," and then explained why. No matter what I asked, he never said anything that was condescending or disingenuous, and he never "pulled rank."

Mostly, he looked bored. The only remark he made was that the air traffic controller was incorrect (after she told us we should deviate from our present heading). After Larry looked at the radar and got on the radio, the controller ultimately agreed with him. When we finally landed for fuel, I looked at him and said, "Who are you, Batman?" He smiled and said, "No, I'm Larry."

To be humble is—knowing your character
and abilities—to be willing to take a lower
place and perform a menial service.

~ Lyman Abbott

As it turns out, Larry Newman was an aviation rock star. He had won the Congressional Gold Medal, awarded by Congress for non-stop flight across the Atlantic Ocean in a balloon. He then flew across the Pacific Ocean in a balloon. He also popularized the sport of hang gliding. In one segment on ABC's *American Sportsman* TV program, he was shown teaching Bob Seagren, a 1968 Olympic Gold medalist in pole vaulting, how to hang glide from the top of a volcano on Maui.

Despite his records, despite his "been there, done that" résumé, he never used his experience to further his purpose, prove a point, or simply tell me to do something without further explanation.

Larry could have gone on and on about all the crazy and amazing things he did in the air. In fact, you could fill books with tales of his antics that, once he felt comfortable with you, he was more than willing to share.

We became fast friends though, at that time, he was dying of pancreatic cancer. He didn't tell me about that either—until I really pressed. I had the amazing fortune to be able to repay the kindness he showed me while flying, by helping him while he was on hospice care.

Larry was an amazing pilot and adventurer. He overcame much in his life on his way to becoming an aviation legend. He wasn't perfect and he had his share of detractors. Despite a few nicks along the way, Larry shined like none other while fulfilling what some may call the menial and mind-numbing boredom that comes as a check pilot. I think being a "check pilot" was Larry's way of giving back to aviation. In that role, he was able to impart some of his encyclopedic knowledge to the next generation of pilots. I'm sure some of the lessons he taught me along the way have saved my life and I'll forever miss him.

OUT IN THE WILD

For our recent book, *Ingredients of Outliers: Women Game Changers*, we interviewed Sharon Guynup, an environmental journalist, photographer, world traveler, and adventurer. At 16, she dropped out of high school to follow a dream born when her grandfather, an amateur photographer, gave her an Instamatic camera when she was five years old.

Her childhood had been a difficult one. Her father was an alcoholic and abusive, and her mother was a sickly woman, addicted to prescription drugs. Guynup ran away from home several times, once landing in a juvenile detention center when her father refused to let her back in their home.

Determined to get an education, she earned her high school equivalency diploma and enrolled in a small local college. It took eight years for Guynup to earn her degree. "I pumped gas, painted houses, wasted away in a cubicle in a brain-numbing job, punched a cash register at a retail store, worked in a ceramics factory, waitressed, and more. But I found a rich life."

Today, Sharon Guynup is a renowned journalist, editor, photographer, and lecturer. She has written on topics ranging from climate change to melting glaciers, fracking, the safety of nanotechnology, the state of the oceans, and animal conservation. Her work has taken her around the world. She's been to the remote heart of Eastern Siberia, to India's Kaziranga National Park, to Turkey's Eastern Anatolian villages, to isolated river towns along Myanmar's Irrawaddy River, across Cuba, to African savannas, and Latin American jungles.

Yet, Guynup has never let success go to her head. In a recent interview, she humbly said: "Looking back on my childhood, I'm grateful there were people along the way at critical points who taught me what I needed to learn, who supported me and helped me get to the next step. So, it's not about feeling proud of myself; it's about feeling really grateful.

"Also, because I've gotten help along the way that helped me create a meaningful career, it's extremely important for me to do the same. I especially like helping kids. When college application season rolls around, I always help a couple of students with their essays and give them ideas on how to apply to school."

To paraphrase John Dickson's definition of humility, Guynup chose "to use her influence for the good of others before herself."

Humble people share the credit and wealth, remaining focused and hungry to continue the journey of success.

~ Rick Pitino

THE "LEVEL 5" LEADER

In his 2001 award-winning and best-selling book, *Good to Great*, Jim Collins studied companies that out-performed the market by a three-fold factor over 15 years. From an initial candidate list of 1,435 companies, "only eleven," he reported, "made the very tough cut into our study." When asked what set those companies apart, Collins and his team concluded that their leaders consistently demonstrate "Level

5" Leadership (his highest rating). He describes the Level 5 leader as "a study in duality: humble and fearless," characterized by two things: steely determination and a culture or attitude of humility.

Great leaders don't need to act tough. Their confidence and humility serve to underscore their toughness.

~ Simon Sinek

Collins goes on to explain how Level 5 leaders respond to the performances of the businesses they lead. When results are poor, the Level 5 leader "looks in the mirror, not out the window, never blaming other people, external factors, or bad luck." When results are good, that same leader "looks out the window, not in the mirror, to apportion credit for the success of the company to other people, external factors, and good luck."

To describe Level 5 leaders, Collins uses the terms:

- "Self-effacing individuals [who] channel their ego needs away from themselves."

- "Compelling modesty—never boastful."

- "Individuals who blend extreme personal humility with intense professional will."

Among those Level 5 leaders profiled in *Good to Great* was a man named Darwin E. Smith who, before being selected CEO of Kimberly-Clark in 1971, had served as its in-house attorney for about a dozen years. Founded in 1872, the paper products company, best-known for Kleenex, had seen its stock fall steadily for 20 years.

Smith's selection surprised nearly everyone; one of the board members even reminded him that he lacked some of the qualifications for leadership. When asked to describe his leadership style, his one-word answer was "eccentric."

In his 20-year tenure as CEO, his bold moves transformed Kimberly-Clark into the world's leading paper-based consumer products company. In each of the last 10 years of his leadership, *Fortune* magazine named it the most admired forest products company in the nation. Yet, Smith remained quietly in the background. He never wrote an autobiography, and was never profiled in a *Wall Street Journal* article.

When asked, upon his retirement, to reveal the secret of his remarkable success, he simply replied, "I never stopped trying to become qualified for the job." Those ten words strike me as an excellent formula for every aspiring self-leader to follow. It's little wonder that in a 2003 *Fortune* article, Collins rated Darwin Smith among the top five "greatest CEOs of all time."

Conversely, in 2009, Collins released a study of once successful companies which had gone in the opposite direction of Kimberly-Clark, and the reasons why. Titled *How the Mighty Fall*, it described such symptoms as: pride born of success, arrogance, complacency with success, loss of focus and passion, and shifting blame to others.

CONTRADICTORY? OR COMPLEMENTARY?

Chances are that, had any of us been asked, out of the blue, what qualities or virtues might best describe such famous outliers as Edmund Hillary or Bill Gates, determination (or self-confidence) would likely have made the list, but I doubt many of us would have included such terms as humble or self-effacing.

The conundrum: If you think you're humble, you likely aren't. Conversely, not thinking yourself humble does *not* somehow confer humility. So, can you demonstrate humility (and believe yourself humble) while, at the same time, demonstrating confidence? Does humility mean passivity, or "to be humbled or humiliated?" Or, is there a more positive way to define it?

In some circles, the word "humility" has taken on more of a negative trait than a positive one. The humble person is portrayed as weak and spineless, an image that perhaps began with a long-ago comic strip titled *The Timid Soul*, featuring a man named Caspar Milquetoast. An older man who could best be described as weak, bland, plain, apologetic, submissive, nondescript, and even cowardly, he was, in every respect, the timid soul.

But do those characteristics even come close to defining humility? Here's John Dickson's answer: "True humility assumes the dignity or strength of the one possessing the virtue, which is why it should not be confused with having low self-esteem or being a doormat for others. In fact, I would go so far as to say that it is impossible to be humble in the real sense without a healthy sense of your own worth and abilities."

In other words, being humble has nothing to do with being walked on, but goes hand in hand with a strong and healthy self-confidence. Not only are the two qualities non-contradictory but they're complementary and most effective when combined. Certainly, no one would ever mistake Bill Gates or Sir Edmund Hillary for Caspar Milquetoast.

Humility is strong, not bold; quiet, not speechless; sure, not arrogant

~ Estelle Smith

CONFIDENT AND CALM

Not long ago, a friend approached me, suffering with what she thought might be a fatal disease. She had muscle wasting in her upper extremities and was getting weaker by the day. These same sort of symptoms could be attributable to a number of ultimately fatal diseases, such as ALS, or Lou Gehrig's disease.

I took her to be examined by a colleague who specializes in that field. After running a series of tests where an electrical current is sent down the extremities to measure the time it takes and a person's reaction to the current, he told her: "You have Thoracic Outlet Syndrome." It's a condition that's unusual for someone her age, so, when I said, "But what about…," he politely cut me off and repeated his diagnosis in a calm and confident manner, without sounding egotistical or contradictory. Although he was assertive, he remained humble in his response.

His humility was evident; he didn't get upset that I had questioned his initial diagnosis. He didn't act threatened, or choose to boast of his many credentials in order to prove he was correct. Rather, his simple, calm, confident response conveyed a level of supreme knowledge and competency, and humility as well. What I learned from him, and from many other encounters, is that confidence doesn't mean arrogance. It simply means you're sure of yourself and are able to convey it in a way that doesn't belittle others.

CONCLUSION

Security and the resultant sense of humility may simply be, as John Dickson said, "to forgo your status…for the good of others before yourself." Thus, security and humility ultimately rest in knowing we're respected and valued by others we respect and value, and whose care and well-being are placed ahead of our own.

In a recent column, Harvey Mackay, best-selling author and business leader, wrote: "Self-confidence alone won't help you succeed, but it's hard to get started or push through the inevitable obstacles without believing in yourself first."

Mackay ended his column with a quote from the late Norman Vincent Peale, author of the classic *The Power of Positive Thinking*: "Believe in yourself. Have faith in your abilities. Without a humble but reasonable belief in your own powers, you cannot be successful or happy."

There you have it—humility and self-confidence—a winning combination!

--- **TAKEAWAYS** ---

- **Be aware** of how often you find yourself talking about yourself to others.

- **Be considerate.** Place the needs of others before your own.

- **Envision everyone** you come into contact with as a teacher. By changing your mindset to one of: "I can learn something from each and every person I encounter," you'll learn more, and quicker than you ever thought possible.

- **Be honest.** It's okay to say, "I don't know the answer to that question." Don't simply guess or make one up. Honesty is respected, as is vulnerability.

- **Be open** to asking for the opinions of co-workers. That may seem like a slower process but, in the end, early collaboration saves time.

- **Learn to listen** more often than you talk during conversations.

- **Laugh** at yourself. Not taking yourself too seriously shows others you realize you're not perfect, and that you're okay learning from your mistakes.

- **Be punctual.** Humble people respect the time of others. By being late, the message you're sending is that your time/schedule/commitments are more important than theirs.

- **When receiving praise, say "thank you" and highlight other members of your team.** Expressing sincere gratitude is a true sign of humility.

2

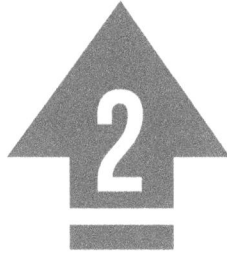

PASSION: SWITCHING TO AFTERBURNER

*You can't be passionate when you feel like it. You have
to be passionate about your job, product or cause all the time.
There's no off switch on a tiger.*

~ Harvey Mackay

Every worthy endeavor is first fueled by passion. Thus, you always hear people say, "Follow your passion!" While it may seem a bit trite, there's a reason that phrase is overused. It's because passion is absolutely everything. Without it, a person merely wanders through life. A life without passion is a life not fully lived and, sadly, usually ends with "If only..."

In saying this, I also acknowledge that there's an incredible amount of pressure put on young women and men to follow their hearts, choose a career path that will fulfill them, and ultimately achieve the goals they set out to achieve.

You may be saying, "How the heck do you figure that out so early in life?" The answer: you don't have to. I'm still discovering new passions. The focus on passion can be overwhelming, and the pressure to choose a path that will fulfill oneself forever isn't always realistic. What the statistics tell us is that you'll likely change college majors and career paths, maybe even a few times—it's all good. My point is that I'm afraid many young people mistake what it means to live a life full of passion with something they need to discover today or, if not today, very soon.

We're told so frequently in life to go "find ourselves," and I think this is part of the problem. For me, the challenge to "go find myself" was confusing—because at the time, I didn't feel all that lost. So, I looked in the mirror—there I was and yet I was no closer to finding myself. Next idea? For the most part, I liked who I was and what I stood for. The general principles I use to guide my life have pretty much stayed the same since I was a young kid.

So what exactly was I supposed to go find? How would I know when I found this ideal version of me that I set out for? It wasn't until I truly sat down and grappled with some of these big questions as a young man that I realized I didn't have to actually find anything. The concept that I needed to go out and look for something meant I wasn't really in control of who I wanted to become. Ultimately, I never did go "find myself." Instead, I *created* myself. I gave myself permission to just be me, and then create the man I wanted to become by—you guessed it—being passionate.

Now, don't get me wrong. I was still realistic about this whole creating myself endeavor. I took stock of who I was, where I was, what my talents and shortcomings were, and then I went from there.

For example, when I was growing up, I loved to play basketball. It was actually more than that—I lived to play basketball. I took a thousand shots a day, and practiced jumping, passing, and dribbling. The challenge was, I simply wasn't very good. I wasn't quick, I had effectively no vertical leap, and little coordination. I used to joke, "Other than that, I could go pro!" Did I have passion for the game? Absolutely! Did my adrenaline pump when I felt that ball in my hands? Yes! (Although that adrenaline came mostly in practice as my main job on game days was to keep the bench nice and warm)

Did I love learning all I could about the game? Of course. Honestly though, I just didn't have the God-given talent needed to be successful at a competitive level. And that's okay. I could've chosen to study broadcasting to become an analyst, or coaching could've been something I poured myself into, but by keeping my mind open, I was able to explore other fields that intrigued me.

A DOCTOR IN THE HOUSE?

My other passion was to care for people by practicing medicine. The challenge here was, unlike basketball, I didn't want to put in the time necessary to pursue good grades. My attitude was always, "When it matters, I will get it done." While I had no problem saying it, there was a nagging feeling in the back of my mind about not being prepared when the time came.

Fortunately, when that time finally did arrive, I had matured enough to figure out how to study. I started the practice, not because I had a true passion for studying, but because I knew medicine was something I loved. First, I needed to get into medical school. Then, I needed to know as much as I could about medicine so I could be the best physician possible. I never wanted to think a patient suffered because of my lack of competence or skill. Not only do I have a heart and a passion for practicing medicine, I'm passionate about challenging myself and competing at the top of my game (even if, at times, I'm only competing against myself).

My mantra has always been: if you can support yourself while pursuing your passion, you have a career. If you can't, you have a hobby. While it's a bit simplistic, it was a good place for me to start narrowing down what I wanted to do. Basketball was, and still is, a hobby of mine. Certainly no one was ever going to pay me to play ball. Medicine, however, is still something I love. Walking into the emergency department energizes me. Not knowing what challenge is going to come in through those doors every day (or night) is exciting. I feel very grateful that, after 30 years, I still love what I do. Thankfully, I got my act together early enough in college so I could actually make something I love into a career.

LET YOUR LIFE SPEAK

Ultimately, and this is the take-home point, I listened to myself. I created what I wanted out of life and did what I needed to do to accomplish my goals. When I graduated near the bottom of my high school class, I'd say I was passionate about sports and having fun. I might not have had a burning desire to excel academically, but I loved life, and I loved people. I still do. What I ultimately chose to do was find an avenue where I could make a living out of my passion for life. I didn't "find myself," I *created* myself. This is the most important point: If I can, you can. I have no special gifts, save passion.

Enough about me. Let's talk about the virtue of living your passion. First, why is pursuing your passion important? The short answer is that it makes life more enjoyable and interesting. It's much easier to spend the time necessary to be great if you love what you're doing. Conversely, life without passion is a life filled with meaningless tasks and unfulfilled dreams.

I think passion in most areas of life is hugely important, whether it's in business, in love, in health, or in medicine. Passion is key. If you have passion, you have this internal drive to succeed. You have this internal want or longing to be better. And so, passion gets you up in the morning. Passion keeps you on your path when you're getting knocked around.

Set yourself earnestly to discover what you are made to do, and then give yourself passionately to the doing of it.
~ Martin Luther King Jr.

I mentor teenagers who want to go to medical school, and I can often tell very early if they're going to make it or not. It's not their grades or their activities or volunteering. It's their body language and the passion in their voice—the "I'd cut off my arm to go to medical school." What I often say to them is, "If you really want to do this and have passion for it, you will do it. Period."

I generally think if you have passion you'll be able to achieve whatever you want, or at least have a great time along the path. Because you will, in fact, be on your path with passion. In order to become a leader, passion is an essential ingredient, an absolute if you want to really be successful at anything.

How do you know when you have it? Let's try and answer that question by taking a look at a few examples of people for whom passion has played a major role in their success.

A LEADER'S LEADER

I can't think of anyone better qualified to address the topic of leadership than John C. Maxwell who, since launching his writing and speaking career in 1995, has become highly respected and widely recognized as a leadership expert. Over the years, organizations he founded, and leads, have trained more than five million leaders around the world.

Maxwell speaks regularly at *Fortune 500* companies, and is a prolific author, with more than 70 books to his credit. Three of his books, *The 21 Irrefutable Laws of Leadership*, *Developing the Leader Within You*, and *The 21 Indispensable Qualities of a Leader*, have each sold more than a million copies. As a result, he was among 25 authors Amazon inducted into its 10th Anniversary Hall of Fame.

In 2014, *Inc.* magazine named Maxwell the top leadership and management expert in the world. His articles on leadership appear regularly in the major business magazines. His column, titled "Maximum Leadership," has long been a monthly feature in *Success* magazine. His photo is on the cover of the magazine's December 2015 issue, and in the lead article, interviewer Josh Ellis describes him as "the world's foremost leadership expert."

Maxwell's newest book, *Intentional Living: Choosing a Life that Matters*, had just been released, and he was asked how he managed to have so much energy at his age (68). "A lot of it is passion," he replied. "If you love what you do and you're helping people, what else would you want to do?"

One of my favorite quotes from Maxwell goes along with that same idea about passion being necessary for everything. "Recently I turned 68," he wrote, "and I am still on fire." He added: "I wake up early, excited to meet the challenges of my day. I'm like a kid. Let me tell you something: You never have to drag a passionate person out of bed!" He offers several tips on how "to fire up your passions." The first is this: "Listen to yourself." He writes: "To tap into your passion, you have to know what you want. Look for clues. What excites you? What makes you dream? What makes your heart sing?"

Unlike his earlier books, Maxwell tells more of his own life story in *Intentional Living*. Asked why he had departed from what had been his typical leadership theme, he said: "Firstly, I think it actually is a leadership book. It's a self-leadership book. The first person you lead should be yourself. And what are leaders? If anything, they're intentional. So I'm saying that you need to get intentional about leading your life. It's not the antithesis of a leadership book. It fits."

Chase down your passion like
it's the last bus of the night.
~ Terri Guillemets

One empowering aspect of being a self-leader, which John Maxwell touches on, is that you're completely and entirely in control of you. You're in complete control of whether or not you're a passionate person; the first person you need to change is yourself. That's so empowering because you don't need anyone else in order to accomplish this goal.

There's no one else who can turn you into a passionate person. But you can.

Read Maxwell's articles. Sit and think about them. Be honest with yourself when you're reflecting. What is it you love so much that you could never give up on? Is it the environment? Animals? Music? Making the world a better place? Chances are, there might be a few things you love so much you could never give up on them. I often say about emergency medicine, "Most days, I'd do it for free; some days they couldn't pay me enough to do it." I suspect I'll practice some form of medicine until the day I die. At some point, in what I hope is the distant future, my body won't be able to handle the rigors of emergency medicine. Hopefully, my mind will be sharp enough that some group, somewhere, needs a volunteer physician!

EXPRESS TO SUCCESS

When Andrew Cherng took out an SBA loan back in 1973 to open a small restaurant in Pasadena, California, there was nothing to suggest it would one day be followed by thousands of other stores and become the dominant chain in its field. At first glance, it may seem like a typical American success story, but this one got its start far away from America.

Cherng, whose given name was Jin Chan Cherng, was born in 1948 in Yangzhou, China. His father was a chef, who moved the family to Taiwan and, several years later, to Japan. His son was a good student, who'd go on to earn a scholarship to Baker University in Kansas and, at the age of 18, immigrate to the United States to enroll. Because he spoke no English, Cherng concentrated on math classes to give him time to learn his new country's language. It was then that he decided to change his first name to Andrew. After earning a bachelor's degree in mathematics, he moved on to the University of Missouri for his master's degree.

Cherng first met his future wife, Peggy Tsiang, at Baker. She was also Chinese, but was born in Burma and raised in Hong Kong. Like

Cherng, Tsiang moved to the U.S. for higher education purposes. After graduating from Baker, she too enrolled at the University of Missouri, and went on to earn a Ph.D. in electrical engineering.

While he was in school, Cherng spent his summer breaks working in New York restaurants. It was there that the first signs of self-leadership began to emerge, as he dreamed of having a restaurant of his own. It would become his lifelong passion.

In 1972, he moved to Los Angeles to help a cousin in the restaurant business, and soon persuaded his family to join him. A year later, his father and he decided to open a sit-down Chinese restaurant in nearby Pasadena, which they named the Panda Inn. Their goal was to feature Mandarin and Szechuan cuisines, rather than the typical Cantonese dishes served in most Chinese restaurants in Southern California.

Peggy Tsiang had also moved to the Los Angeles area, where she put her engineering skills to work on large government contracts at such giant companies as 3M and McDonnell Douglas. Tsiang and Cherng were married in 1975 and, when Cherng's father died several years later, Tsiang joined the family business on a full-time basis.

IN THE FAST LANE

The restaurant grew in popularity, but Andrew Cherng had a bigger dream, and began looking for a good location to open a second Panda Inn. In a meeting with the developers of the brand new Glendale Galleria shopping center, they suggested he consider opening a quick-serve location in its food court. That marked the birth of Panda Express in 1983. Within two years, there were nine stores, all in area shopping malls. The Cherngs quickly recognized the need to add stand-alone stores and, by 1993, they owned and operated one hundred facilities, with combined annual sales exceeding $2 billion.

Today, the still privately held Panda Restaurant Group consists of more than 1,800 restaurants and 27,000 employees all across the United States and in Mexico, South Korea, and Dubai. Andrew and Peggy Cherng, now in their late sixties, remain co-CEOs, with

Andrew the visionary and motivator, and Peggy the operations wizard. Along the way, these two immigrants, who came with nothing and spoke no English, have amassed a personal fortune estimated at more than $3 billion.

Their success has brought the Cherngs wide recognition in the Chinese-American community. For example, in 2000, Andrew was invited to join the prestigious Committee of 100, a membership organization of Chinese Americans founded in 1990, and "dedicated to the spirit of excellence and achievement in America." Members of this elite by-invitation-only group include such world-renowned figures as architect I.M. Pei, cellist Yo-Yo Ma, YouTube co-founder Steve Chen, and figure skating champion Michelle Kwan.

The Committee of 100's website notes the role passion has played in Andrew Cherng's life: "What started as a passion for food has evolved into a passion for life, learning and people. Whether improving the front-of-store experience or creating career paths for his associates, Andrew is known to encourage and inspire people to better themselves personally and professionally. The company embraces a core purpose to bring out the best in each associate and develop their capabilities—a direct result of Andrew's passion for personal growth."

Passion transcends languages, borders and cultures, and is an important quality for every self-leader to have.

Buried deep within each of us is a spark of greatness,
a spark than can be fanned into flames of
passion and achievement. That spark is not
outside of you; it is born deep within you.

~ James A. Ray

OTHERWISE IMPOSSIBLE TASKS

Easton LaChappelle was participating in a Colorado science fair in 2011 when he noticed a seven-year-old girl with a prosthetic hand. It was a simple device that could only open and close, so he was astounded when her parents told him it had cost them $80,000. Worse still, she would soon outgrow it, and need a replacement. LaChappelle was confident he could do better. A curious 14-year-old, he'd begun taking things apart when he was eight. From toys to toasters, kitchen appliances to electronic gadgets, he was determined to discover all he could about them.

He'd moved on to robotics and managed to put together a prosthetic hand, using Lego blocks, fishing wire, and some electrical tubing. It wasn't exactly high-tech, but it worked. Before long, LaChappelle developed a system of making prosthetic limbs using a 3-D printer. The robotic hand he'd shown at the science fair received a third-place award. Thus, his chance meeting with that little girl convinced him he could make a better device at a fraction of the cost. His goal: to make one for less than a thousand dollars.

Every great dream begins with a dreamer. Always remember, you have within you the strength, the patience and the passion to reach for the stars to change the world.

~ Harriet Tubman

That was four years ago. Today, 19-year-old LaChappelle is the CEO of a company he founded. Unlimited Tomorrow, Inc. points clearly to the direction in which this passionate young self-leader is headed. Its mission statement includes these words: "enabling humans to perform otherwise impossible tasks."

LaChappelle's passion is clearly demonstrated in all he does. Having perfected his low-cost prosthetic arm, with the help of several colleagues and significant input from amputees, he has made the software for it available on an open source basis, meaning it can be downloaded and used by anyone, at no cost.

But he's just getting started, with a focus not only on prosthetic limbs but on the body as a whole. LaChappelle is leading his team at Unlimited Tomorrow in developing a new concept of an exoskeleton that will help paraplegics walk again. There are some exoskeletons available today, but they're primarily worn externally and tend to be cumbersome and costly. LaChappelle's vision is for one that can be ordered inexpensively online, be quickly and easily donned, and worn undetected beneath the clothes, giving the wearer the freedom to once again perform what had long been "otherwise impossible tasks."

For this passionate young man, there really is an "unlimited tomorrow."

HUNGRY TO LEARN

In *Outliers in Law*, part of our series featuring inspirational men and women who excel in their chosen fields, we tell the story of attorney Sarah Buel. Buel is currently a Clinical Professor of Law at the Sandra Day O'Connor College of Law at Arizona State University and a well-known advocate for battered women and abused children.

Her passion for the victims of domestic violence has taken her on a long and often difficult journey that began many years ago, when she herself was victimized by a violent, alcoholic husband. It was a journey that would take her from New York to New Hampshire, back to New York, then to California, Massachusetts, Colorado, Washington, Massachusetts (again), Texas and eventually to Arizona.

In 1977, with her two-year-old son, Buel left her husband and began to follow what had been her dream since childhood—to become a lawyer, one who would dedicate her life to fighting for victims of domestic violence.

Buel had little going for her. She was 12 when her parents divorced and, rather than take sides, she moved away, living a nomadic existence that included attending eight different high schools. When she divorced her husband, she was living in New York with little money and a baby to raise. However, Buel was able to enroll in a federal training program, where she learned of an opening for a paralegal position with the Legal Aid Society—in New Hampshire.

The odds were long. A number of the applicants had college degrees, so she told the interviewer: "I know I only have a high school diploma, but I'll fight harder than anybody else. And I'm so hungry to learn."

That hunger paid off, and Buel was able to gain valuable experience in setting up and overseeing the state's first battered women's shelters, and helping write new abuse prevention legislation. At the same time, she was determined to take the next step, which meant a college degree. Buel applied at several universities and, when offered a scholarship to Columbia, she returned to New York to accept it.

She did well there but, for personal safety reasons, decided to leave New York. Offered a scholarship to Stanford, Buel drove across the country with her young son, only to be told a mistake had been made and she would get no financial aid. Hearing that Harvard operated an extension school in Cambridge, she called and was offered a grant. Back she drove and began night classes there, with detours to Denver and Seattle, eventually earning a bachelor's degree, one that had taken her seven years and thousands of miles to obtain.

With diploma in hand, Buel applied to Harvard Law School, despite warnings that she was wasting her time, that "you're not the Harvard type." Proving how wrong her naysayers were, she was not only admitted but was granted a full scholarship. That was in 1987 and, three years later, she graduated *cum laude*!

My mission in life is not merely to survive, but to thrive; and to do so with some passion, some compassion, some humor, and some style.

~ Maya Angelou

Sarah Buel is a colleague of mine at the Sandra Day O'Connor College of Law. Passion literally oozes from her pores. I'd never want to oppose her in court on any issue she's committed to winning.

For 37 years, Buel has been a leader in the fight to eliminate domestic violence, and to defend and protect its victims. Along the way, she has received frequent recognition and numerous awards. Here's a brief sampling:

- Received the American Bar Association's *Top Twenty Young Lawyers Award* (1992)

- Narrated the Academy-Award winning documentary, *Defending Our Lives* (1992)

- Named one of the five most inspiring women in America by NBC (1996)

- Received the ASU Centennial Professor Award (2013)

- Received the American Bar Association's 20/20 Vision Award (2015)

Recently asked about the role passion has played in her life, she replied: "Oh, absolutely, I'm passionate about this work. One of my greatest hopes is to inspire my students to be champions for social justice, hoping it becomes their life work. I'm doing what I love and following my passion. I have a sense of mission that I'm here to do this work."

CONCLUSION

I have passion, passion in a lot of areas and for many things. It's a blessing and a curse, inasmuch as I don't take or require much true down time because I'm generally busy doing things I love to do. Thus, getting up early (or staying up late) has never been a challenge. In fact, every morning, I leap out of bed as if on afterburner.

For years, I lived by the following motto "wake up, be kind, kick ass!" This is not difficult when you have passion. The take-home point is this: find your passion. Likely you have many passions and all it takes is some courage and self-exploration to open the door to your future. What are you waiting for? Find that fire within you. Get it done!

───────────────── **TAKEAWAYS** ─────────────────

- **Figure out** what gets you excited to jump out of bed in the morning; then figure out how to make it your avocation or hobby.

- **Learn** everything you can about what excites you, and about those who excel pursuing it.

- **Plot and pilot your own course,** knowing you'll make lots of minor and sometimes major course corrections along the way. By the way, the fun is in the corrections.

- **Find internships,** or professionals who'll allow you to job shadow them. Passionate people demonstrate their enthusiasm my helping others.

- **Surround yourself** with other passionate people. Avoid negativity, and pessimistic people; they're destructive.

- **Make a list** of the top ten reasons you're doing what you're doing. Tape it to the back of your medicine cabinet. Sometimes, after a long day, being reminded why you're here in the first place definitely helps!

- **Start each day** by thinking of three things you're excited to conquer that day.

- **Don't be afraid** to change direction. Just because something once excited you doesn't mean it always will. And that's okay. Nothing worthwhile was ever discovered in a straight line.

- **Speak with conviction.** People should be able to hear passion in your voice. Would you follow someone who lacked passion for a cause?

CHAPTER

3

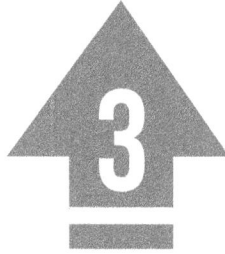

INTEGRITY: A FOREVER VALUE

*If I could teach only one value to live by, it would be this:
Success will come and go, but integrity is forever. Integrity
means doing the right thing at all times and in all circumstances,
whether or not anyone is watching.*

~ Amy Rees Anderson

Amy Rees Anderson is, among other things, an award-winning author, speaker, entrepreneur and the founder and CEO of REES Capital, an angel investment and advising firm based in South Jordan, Utah. Its name reflects its mission: "Recognizing and Empowering Entrepreneurial Success."

Prior to launching REES Capital, Anderson was the founder and CEO of MediConnect Global, Inc., a worldwide leader in medical record retrieval, digitization, and one of the largest cloud-based health information exchanges. She led all aspects of MediConnect's business, including a worldwide workforce of more than a thousand employees. Under her direction, the company achieved over 1500 percent growth. In March 2012, she successfully sold MediConnect for more than $377 million.

An active angel investor, Anderson recently founded the IPOP Foundation, a charity focused on helping educate and mentor entrepreneurs. She's also a regular contributor to *Forbes* magazine and *The Huffington Post*. The quote I used to introduce this chapter was the opening sentence of an article published in *Forbes* on November 28, 2012. In the opening paragraph, she adds this warning: "Building a reputation of integrity takes years, but it takes only a second to lose, so never allow yourself to ever do anything that would damage your integrity."

Simply put, integrity is doing what you say and saying what you'll do—whether or not anyone is watching. The term is derived from the Latin word *integer*, which means "whole or complete." When a person has integrity, he or she is believed to have an inner sense of "wholeness," derived from consistency of action and character. The characteristics or qualities that comprise integrity are often defined as truthfulness, honesty, consistency, morality, accountability, responsibility, and loyalty.

To me, integrity means always doing what is right and good, regardless of the immediate consequences. It means being righteous from the very depth of our soul, not only in our actions but, more importantly, in our thoughts and in our hearts.

~ Joseph B. Wirthlin

Then there are those instances when a revered role model decides something a bit out of character is okay, "just this once." Sadly, we hear these morale crushing stories in the headlines nearly every week. We hear so many of them that I don't want to give negativity too much power as a motivating factor, but it's important for every leader to know your integrity can be gone in a minute. Although this truth is overwhelming and a bit terrifying, it's an important fact to always keep in the forefront of your mind. Becoming—and remaining—a woman or man of integrity is not always easy. It isn't always fun, either.

Some of the most difficult decisions I've made are the ones of which I'm most proud. They weren't easy to make, and there was a bit of discomfort that came along with missing a supposed opportunity, but being able to look at the long-term outcome and feel proud is powerful.

As self-leaders, you ultimately answer to you. If you cut corners, stretch the truth, or mislead others, even if no one else ever knows, you will. Trust me: doing the right thing always feels better than the alternative in the end. As motivational author and speaker Zig Ziglar said, "With integrity, you have nothing to fear, since you have nothing to hide. With integrity, you will do the right thing, so you will have no guilt."

It's important to note that choosing integrity over the alternative has its side benefits. Striving to be a man of integrity has served me well in my relationships. By saying what I mean and doing what I say, others can trust that I'll be consistent with my word, and honor my commitments, no matter the outcome.

WHERE IT BEGINS

Ideally, integrity training starts in the home and it starts early. With kids at home, you never have to wonder "whether or not anyone is watching." You can be sure you're being watched all the time. As the late Dr. Roy L. Smith cautioned: "We tend to forget that children watch examples better than they listen to preaching."

My wife René and I are very proud of our son Michael and his younger sister Kaleigh. Their actions almost always reflect their intentions. They're often the ones I use as a barometer for my own sincerity.

René is the reason we're blessed with such fantastic kids. She modeled her values and integrity day in and day out during their formative years. Today, they're the kind of individuals I wanted to be at their respective ages.

Don't get me wrong; they're not perfect angels. However, when they do screw up—as we all do—they're the first to call themselves out, repair what needs repairing, and then move on. It's remarkable how fearless they both are at giving and receiving constructive criticism.

"OWNING IT"

For example, my son Michael is a member of the Air National Guard. Currently, he's going through fighter pilot training. This consists of flying progressively advanced planes in progressively difficult situations. The Air Force demands perfection. He recently told me that if you're even a few feet off the assigned altitude or airspeed, you'll end up on the receiving end of a painful, one-way conversation.

Michael's always been good at "owning it," but I wondered how he'd react to someone yelling in his face. Neither René nor I ever raised our voices. In fact, when I needed to have a direct conversation with them, I'd *lower* my voice and talk slowly. So I wasn't sure what effect being screamed at from close range would have.

When I asked him, he responded, "They wouldn't yell if I hadn't screwed up. In the Air Force, the only acceptable action is to take responsibility, not make excuses, and do it right the next time—that simple." As you can imagine, I couldn't have been more proud of him. There was no ego involved, just honest pragmatism.

Kaleigh's the same way. When she approached me about starting a business, it was all I could do to not jump in and do it with her. In fact, I tried to help, even knowing this was something she had to do for herself. I simply couldn't help myself. Yet she shut me down immediately. "Dad, you know I have to figure this part out on my own so that I really know it…" and my own words were gently fed back to me.

Kaleigh's incredibly capable and knows herself very well, and she knew she had to be the one who took the necessary steps to get her venture up and running. Another amazing quality she has is that she doesn't talk ill of anyone.

RENÉ'S ROLE

As a physician who works in hospice, René is a compassionate, caring professional who helps people during some of the most difficult times of their existence. She not only cares for her dying patients, but offers support and guidance for their families as well. I know her experiences in the field of hospice have bubbled over into our collective daily life. She has continually instilled in us the mantra that "We each have our own reality." So, she would say, "If you don't know where others are coming from, how can you really judge their behavior?"

This mindset has made life, particularly practicing medicine, much more enjoyable for me. After finally getting my own head around it, I stopped trying to impose my values or beliefs on others. Instead of acting as an arbitrator for "healthy living," I became a coach if someone wanted one. If they didn't, no problem, I was still there to assist them in their current situation. What could be easier than that?

My "takeaways" from René and my children are simple, yet often difficult to master completely. Don't judge, accept responsibility, don't talk ill of people behind their back, and always try your hardest; it might be your last chance.

The supreme quality for leadership is unquestionably integrity. Without it, no real success is possible, no matter whether it is on a section gang, a football field, in an army, or in an office.
~ Dwight D. Eisenhower

THE PEOPLE'S BANKER

The son of Italian immigrants, he was born in 1870 in San Jose, California. When he was seven, his father died and, at age 14, he decided to drop out of school and go to work for his stepfather, who was in the produce business. He performed so well that, within five years, he'd become a full partner. At age 31, this young self-leader sold his interest to company employees, and decided to retire. It was 1901, marking the dawn of the 20th century, in which he would have a significant impact.

But Amadeo Pietro Giannini wouldn't stay retired for very long. He had already developed a reputation as a man of integrity and was invited to join the board of directors of the Columbia Savings and Loan Society, a small bank in a section of San Francisco called "Little Italy." In those days, most banks, including this one, catered to the needs of the well-known and the wealthy. But A.P., as he was best known, was more concerned about the needs of those he called the "little fellows," the working people and small business owners who comprised most of the community.

Giannini tried unsuccessfully to persuade bank officials to change their policies to accommodate the working class, and, in 1904, he resigned. With the help of some friends, he raised $150,000 and opened a new bank in the community, which he named the Bank of Italy. From the beginning, he made it clear what his mission was. "A banker," he said, "should consider himself a servant of the people, a servant of the community. This is my role; this is me and what I want to do; and I am convinced I can do it."

Integrity is the first step to true greatness ... To maintain it in high places costs self-denial; in all places it is liable to opposition, but its end is glorious, and the universe will yet do it homage.

~ Charles Simmons

Giannini was unwavering in his commitment. In 1906, when a major earthquake devastated San Francisco, forcing the closure of the city's banks, he was the first to take action. A wooden plank, sitting atop two barrels on the street outside his bank, became his new "office," and he began making loans based solely on what he described as "a man's face and a signature." Years later, he would report that every one of those loans had been repaid in full.

That experience made him more determined than ever to make banking services available to everyone—not just the well-known and wealthy. He began by opening branch offices of his bank, an unheard of practice in the industry at that time, and derided by other bankers. Within a decade, however, Bank of Italy had two dozen branches and had become California's fourth largest bank. That number would later grow to more than 500 branches and, in 1929, Giannini combined it with other banks he had acquired; thus Bank of America was born.

In 1930, he retired for the second time, convinced he had left his bank in good hands. However, as the Great Depression began taking its toll, the bank's new leaders decided to start selling some of its branches. Feeling betrayed, Giannini waged a successful campaign to regain control and again took on active leadership of the bank. During the campaign, he wrote in a note to his son, "It's right and principle we are battling for, and there's no compromise with right or principle, regardless of consequences. No sir, never, my boy."

By the time he retired for the third and final time in 1945, Bank of America had become the nation's largest financial institution, known simply in many circles as "B of A."

In 1949, A.P. Giannini, a man of vision and unswerving integrity, died. But his role in revolutionizing the banking industry around the world continued to be recognized. Several buildings in California bear his name and *Time* magazine hailed him among "the builders and titans" of the 20th century. He was the only banker included in the prestigious *Time 100* list and, in 2010, his name was added to the California Hall of Fame.

WHO IS THIS GUY?

Those four words were emblazoned on the cover of the October 18, 1999 cover of *Sports Illustrated*, which also featured a large photo of a

National Football League quarterback who, after the first four games of that season, had already thrown 14 touchdown passes in leading his team to four straight victories. They were not only his first four games as an NFL starter, but his prior experience in the league included a grand total of four passes completed in 11 attempts, for a combined 39 yards! No wonder the magazine asked who he was.

The questions soon stopped, as Kurt Warner would go on to stardom during a 12-year NFL career, first with the St. Louis Rams and then, after a brief stint with the New York Giants, the Arizona Cardinals. He'd played quarterback in high school and college with some success but not enough to be drafted by any NFL teams. After getting his degree in 1994, he had a couple of tryouts but it wasn't until 1998 that the Rams signed him to his first NFL contract—as the third-string quarterback.

The high road is always respected. Honesty
and integrity are always rewarded.

~ Scott Hamilton

As the 1999 season began, injuries to other players forced the Rams to name Warner as the starting quarterback, and the team was projected to finish the season in last place. Instead, he led the Rams to a 13-3 regular season record and on to victory in the Super Bowl. As a result, Warner was named the NFL's Most Valuable Player of the season, and of the Super Bowl as well. Two years later, he was again named the league's Most Valuable Player, and led the Rams to its second Super Bowl appearance in a three-year span.

In 2005, after one year with the New York Giants, Warner joined the Arizona Cardinals, where he continued his outstanding career. In 2008, the team won its first division title in a decade, followed by its first appearance in the Super Bowl. After leading the Cardinals to the playoffs again the following season, he announced his retirement. To this day, he's considered the best undrafted player in National Football League history.

FIRST THINGS FIRST

But the Kurt Warner story is about a lot more than football. He not only excelled as a player but has stood out as a man of integrity. Not long after graduating from college, and having his efforts to become an NFL player rebuffed, Warner took a job stocking shelves at a local grocery store, making $5.50 per hour. He'd recently met an attractive young woman named Brenda who was going through difficult times. She was a Marine veteran and single mom with two children, one of whom had suffered a serious accident, leaving him brain-damaged and blind.

While such circumstances might have deterred most single young men from pursuing a deeper relationship, Warner's response was completely the opposite. The love and compassion he showed, both to Brenda and her kids, convinced her he was the man for her. They married in 1997 and Warner adopted the children. Since then, the Warners have had five more children.

As Kurt Warner's NFL career took off in 1999, he and his wife launched the Kurt Warner First Things First Foundation. The foundation is dedicated to impacting lives by promoting their Christian values, sharing, experiencing, and providing opportunities to encourage everyone that anything is possible when people seek to "put first things first." The "first things" they refer to are faith and family. The foundation has been involved in such worthwhile causes as children's hospitals, people with developmental disabilities, and assisting single parents.

Kurt Warner's achievements, as player, husband, father, athlete, humanitarian, and philanthropist, have been well recognized. In 2008, he received the NFL's Walter Payton Man of the Year Award, given each year to a player in recognition of his charitable and volunteer activities, in addition to his excellence on the field. In 2009, *USA Weekend* named him the winner of its annual Most Caring Athlete

Award and, in a poll of National Football League players by *Sports Illustrated*, he was chosen as the league's best role model, both on and off the field.

Beginning in 1989, the Athletes in Action/Bart Starr Award has been presented annually to the NFL player who best exemplifies outstanding character and leadership in the home, on the field, and in the community. Representatives from each of the 32 NFL teams, plus all former winners of the award, staff members of the Athletes in Action ministry, and Bart Starr himself, submit nominations, with the winner announced during Super Bowl festivities. In presenting the 2010 award to Kurt Warner, Starr commented: "We have never given this award to anyone more deserving."

A PRESCRIPTION FOR INTEGRITY

In our recently published book, *Outliers in Medicine*, we profiled a woman named Angela Nuzzarello, who has been a pioneer in the field of medical education for many years. Doctor Nuzzarello holds both an M.D. degree and a Master's Degree in Health Professions Education (MPHE). She is currently Associate Dean of Student Affairs and Associate Professor of Psychiatry at the Oakland University William Beaumont School of Medicine in Rochester, Michigan. During her career, she has earned multiple awards for her contributions to medical education.

In our interview, we asked her what advice she'd offer to those who might want to follow in her footsteps:

"First, don't compromise. If you're going to be successful you have to be who you are, and you can't compromise who you are or your values, in order to be successful in any environment.

"Second, always do more than is expected of you. One of the reasons I was successful early on in my career was that I always did so. If someone said, 'I need you to work on this or do this,' I'd do it and then I'd think, 'Okay, what else? What could I do to make this a little bit different or a little bit better?' You know, that extra push.

"Also, appreciate the people who make you look good on a daily basis. Anybody who's successful has so many people around—whether it's family members or co-workers. There are many people who make me look good much of the time. It's important to make sure you appreciate those people and let them know how much value there is in what they do.

"The last thing is about being dependable and trying to figure out how you can lighten someone else's load. That's always appreciated when you're not centered on yourself, but also thinking about what you can do for someone else."

There we have it: don't compromise, go the extra mile, appreciate others, be dependable. To me, that sounds like an excellent prescription for integrity.

I've heard this C.S. Lewis quote many times through my life, and it seems to be a guiding principle in Dr. Nuzzarello's life; "Integrity is doing what is right, even when no one else is watching."

"Integrity, like humility, is a quality which vanishes the moment we are conscious of it in ourselves. We see it only in others."
~ Madeleine L'Engle

CONCLUSION

Integrity is both easy and hard. It can be hard when no one's looking and the stakes are high, and yet those times are the most rewarding when you "nail it." On a day to day basis, most of us are not challenged to any great degree on high stakes issues and it's relatively easy to stay on track.

The key is to practice having integrity on the small things. So when you are really tested, your compass never wavers and you stay the course. When you look in the mirror at the end of the day, be proud of the person looking back.

TAKEAWAYS

- **Evaluate** your behavior at the end of every day. Did you demonstrate integrity in both your words and actions?

- **Ask yourself** the hard questions. Where have you fallen short and what can you do to improve your actions?

- **Keep promises** you make. The ones you make to yourself are just as important as the ones you make to others.

- **Don't gossip.** People are much less likely to trust you if they hear you speaking negatively about another person, even if they might agree with you. Keep any negative talk to yourself.

- **Don't whine,** or place blame on other people or situations. Accept responsibility for your actions. If you're the common denominator of all your problems, the fix is easy—you.

- **Keep secrets** when someone chooses to confide in you. Honor that person by doing so. Continue proving your trustworthiness.

- **Be true** to yourself. Don't feel you need to share everything with everyone in order to be a person of integrity. If you're asked a question you feel uncomfortable answering, it's okay to respond with, "I appreciate you asking, but I'd rather not answer that question," or "I'm not at liberty to discuss that right now." This is still an example of honesty.

- **Follow through.** You are what you do, not what you say you'll do.

- **Look** people in the eyes when you talk to them, especially when making promises. In many cultures, avoiding eye contact is seen as a sign that you might be hiding something.

CHAPTER

4

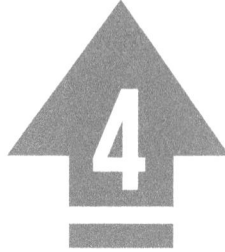

LEARNING: THERE'S WISDOM IN THE WHYS

*From the dawn of time, whenever humanity has wanted to
know more, we have achieved it most effectively not by
removing ourselves from the world to ponder and theorize,
but rather by getting our hands dirty and making careful observations
of real stuff. In short, we have learned primarily by tinkering.*

~ Curt Gabrielson

Both as noun and verb, the word *tinker* has been part of our language for centuries. However, until recently, the word has primarily been defined in, at best, a neutral way or, more often, in a negative one. In any case, it's not a word one would have chosen to describe himself or herself during a job interview or on a résumé.

As a noun, the word originally described a person who wandered from place to place mending pots and pans, and other metal kitchen items. It was mostly downhill from there, used to describe a clumsy worker, a bungler, a meddler, a time waster, or a gypsy. As a verb, it typically meant to work in an unskilled, clumsy, and/or useless way. To *tinker* would certainly not have been seen as having an effective role in the learning process.

So it strikes me as rather ironic that in the rapidly changing, explosive, disruptive, and innovative age in which we live, and with the world's knowledge literally at our fingertips, this ancient word has taken on a new and very respectable reputation. *Tinker* is now a part of a growing awareness of the need to provide broader and more flexible learning opportunities for everyone.

Curt Gabrielson is an educator and author, whose book, *Tinkering: Kids Learn by Making Stuff,* was released in 2013. A graduate of the prestigious Massachusetts Institute of Technology (MIT), he writes: "While I did learn a good bit at MIT, what I learned on the hog farm of my youth turned out to be much more applicable to life." In a recent blog post, he adds: "I've criticized official curricula for as long as I can remember. I scorned silly memorization in my high school chemistry class. I raised my eyebrows at the esoteric content of required mathematics courses in college."

I'm a tinkerer, so I can relate to Gabrielson's feelings and perhaps you can as well. I've worn a lot of different hats during my career. Not all of them fit—in retrospect, some looked ridiculous, but it was the act of tinkering itself that taught me the most.

It started early. When I was five, I built an "elevator" in my basement out of a tin coffee can, a bushel basket, a rope, and a large rock. I stood in the bushel basket that was tied to the coffee can suspended by the rope, which was then strung over a nail about six feet above the floor. I lifted the rock up and tossed it into the can, expecting the change in weight distribution to propel me skyward. Instead, the coffee can containing the large rock came crashing down on my head. As opposed to me shooting skyward, the event propelled me into the emergency department, resulting in five sutures, a bald spot, and my first encounter with emergency medicine.

Never stop learning. Whether you are an entry-level employee fresh from college or a CEO, you don't know it all. Admitting this is not a sign of weakness. The strongest leaders are those who are lifelong learners.

~ Indra Nooyi

Undaunted, I continue to try new things, or new ways of doing old things. Often, I end up bruised or cut, as when I was five. Nevertheless, I'd do it all again. Knowledge is transferable. Lessons I learned from making an elevator, or flying, or running a hot dog stand, transfer to other businesses and careers. Back in the day, my classmates and I dreamed of the time when we'd complete our formal education and could get on with living! We were ready for the time when we could take all learning we'd accumulated and put it to work, providing some return on those years we'd spent in classrooms.

That said, walking across the stage and accepting a diploma was always bittersweet for me. In some ways, I couldn't wait to get out and change the world. In others, I loved the protection of the classroom and academia. But I finally realized that if you're wise, the learning process shouldn't stop the day you bid the campus farewell. That diploma or degree may testify that you've been educated, but education and wisdom aren't the same thing, nor are education and learning synonymous.

Oftentimes, the very concept of education and learning is troublesome. When I write the word "learning" or "education," my guess is that it may conjure up some image of a stereotypical student, a desk, and a paper and pencil. In order to be the best self-leader you can be, you need to create a new learning paradigm. Rethink education. Rethink learning. Rethink the concept of the teacher teaching, and the student silently absorbing information.

To be clear, I'm a true believer in education, formal and informal. I love the times I've been able to sit in classrooms and soak up knowledge.

That being said, I also acknowledge the incredible amount of truly life-changing learning experiences I've had outside the classroom, such as traveling, interacting with patients and colleagues, starting new ventures, succeeding, and especially knowledge gained from failing.

I set a goal decades ago to go back to school every ten years. I've been fortunate that I've been able to stick with this, and it has changed my life. However, I also say that having an open concept in regard to learning has made all the difference in the world. Learning and growth don't just happen in isolation inside a classroom. When you open your mind to this truth, the world becomes your classroom, and life itself becomes your ever-present, enduring teacher.

THE CURIOSITY GENE

Our curiosity gene shows up early in life, as any parent can testify. I can still hear the sound of my two little children's voices saying "why." Here's a good description making the rounds on Twitter and Facebook, "A child is an island of curiosity surrounded by a sea of question marks." Children have an innate desire to learn about the world and the way it works. As relentless as the "whys" can seem, this desire needs to be fostered and supported. Truth be told, as exhausting as it might have been to answer their questions, I never wanted my children's inquiring minds to stop seeking answers.

The great ancient Greek philosopher Socrates understood that the four-year-old really has it right in terms of learning. Socrates knew the best way to learn was to question everything, and to continue asking questions in order to deeply understand life and the world in which we live.

The 17th century English philosopher and physician John Locke called curiosity "an appetite after knowledge." Twenty-four centuries after Socrates, American psychiatrist and teacher Smiley Blanton described it as "nature's original school of education." In his 1986 book, *Made in*

Japan, Akio Morita, co-founder of SONY Corporation, called it "the key to creativity."

To Robert MacNeil, Canadian-American novelist, journalist, and former TV personality, curiosity is "the most basic human trait," and Anne Sweeney, former president of the Disney Channel and current Netflix board member, says: "curiosity leads to new ideas, new jobs, new industries." Clearly, the importance of curiosity as a key to learning has long been acknowledged and recognized all around the world.

CURIOSITY ISLAND

I recently finished reading a new book titled *A Curious Mind: The Secret to a Bigger Life*. It's basically a self-portrait, written and told by Brian Grazer, assisted by journalist and author Charles Fishman. If you're a movie buff, Grazer's name may be familiar to you. For many years, he's been one of Hollywood's most successful producers, whose screen credits include *The Da Vinci Code, American Gangster, 8 Mile, A Beautiful Mind*, and many more.

Grazer isn't just the king of the big screen; he's been involved in a slew of successful TV shows as well: *24, Empire, Arrested Development,* and *Friday Night Lights*, just to name a few. His films and TV shows have been nominated for 43 Academy Awards and 149 Emmys—so far! In 2007, *Time* included his name on its list of the "100 Most Influential People in the World."

Grazer dedicated the book to his grandmother, writing: "Starting when I was a boy, she treated every question I asked as valuable. She taught me to think of myself as curious, a gift that has served me every day of my life."

Indeed, Grazer has spent his life on a proverbial Curiosity Island, conducting what he calls "Curiosity Conversations" with people in nearly every field of endeavor, asking them about their lives and their work. His book includes a list of several hundred people with whom he's visited: athletes and astronauts, cops and crooks, presidents and prime ministers, scientists and skateboarders, TV personalities and tattoo artists, Olympic gold medalists and Pulitzer Prize winners.

Grazer began his career as a law clerk for an attorney at the famous Warner Bros. Studios in 1974. He got the job after overhearing a conversation by two young men outside his apartment window. One mentioned that he'd just quit his job and named the employer. His curiosity aroused, Grazer looked up the phone number, made a call, was interviewed the following day, and was immediately hired. "At that moment," he writes, "I had found my life's work. ... I joined the world of show business. I never again worked at anything else."

Learn from others. Ask questions. Be a good listener.
Get a pulse beat of what is going on around you.
~ Paul "Bear" Bryant

In telling that story, he said: "My kind of curiosity hasn't changed much since I eavesdropped on those guys at my apartment complex. It hasn't actually changed that much since I was an antsy twelve-year-old boy. ... Curiosity has been the most valuable quality, the most important resource, the central motivation of my life. I think curiosity should be as much a part of our culture, our educational system, and our workplaces, as concepts like 'creativity' and 'innovation.'"

In his view, however, that's not the case. "The classroom," he writes, "should be a vineyard of questions, a place to cultivate them, to learn both how to ask them and how to chase down the answers ... but authentic curiosity in a typical seventh-grade classroom isn't cultivated—because it's inconvenient and disruptive to the orderly running of the class."

As for our workplaces, Grazer cites a 2011 case study in *Harvard Business Review* about the innovation and creativity endeavors of Proctor & Gamble. He points out that, in that 5,000-word article, "innovation" is used 65 times, while "curiosity" is never mentioned.

"That's crazy," he laments. "We simply don't credit curiosity. We don't even credit curiosity when we're using it, describing it, and extolling it."

Given the apparent lack of emphasis on curiosity in the workplace or the classroom, how then does the budding self-leader learn that important skill? According to Grazer, it's basically a do-it-yourself endeavor. "Curiosity is a state of mind," he insists. "More specifically, it's the state of having an open mind. Curiosity is a kind of receptivity. And best of all, there is no trick to curiosity. You just have to ask one good question a day, and listen to the answer. ... It is, truly, the secret to living a bigger life."

> *I happen to be a kind of inquisitive guy and when I see things I don't like, I start thinking why do they have to be like this and how can I improve them?*
>
> ~ Walt Disney

THE MAKER MOVEMENT

Tinkering, of course, is a classic example of curiosity in action. The foreword of the earlier mentioned Gabrielson's book was written by Dale Dougherty, founder and CEO of California-based Maker Media, Inc., the producer of *Maker* magazine and Maker Faire. Described as "part science fair, county fair, and part something entirely new, Maker Faire is an all-ages gathering of tech enthusiasts, crafters, educators, tinkerers, hobbyists, engineers, science clubs, authors, artists, students, and commercial exhibitors. All of these 'makers' come to Maker Faire to show what they have made and to share what they have learned."

Launched in 2006, the Maker Faires have expanded rapidly. Eight years after the inaugural event, 215,000 people, half of them children, attended its two flagship events, in the San Francisco Bay Area and New York. That same year, more than one hundred independently produced faires were held in cities around the world.

According to its website, "A worldwide Maker Movement is transforming innovation in industry, hands-on learning in education and the personal lives of makers of all ages."

In *Tinkering*, Dougherty writes: "Formal learning often doesn't make sense without informal learning. It offers too much theory without enough grounding in practice. Tinkering represents this kind of practical education that is often undervalued in formal settings."

He adds: "I believe that today's children are demanding such learning experiences because they know how essential it is for them to grow as learners and become creative contributors to society."

He concludes with this question: "If we can get more of us tinkering, who knows what tough problems we can solve, what discoveries we will find and what new things we will create?"

In response, Gabrielson writes: "What you want to see happen is thoughtful tinkering. You want to see kids thinking about what they're tinkering with. I assume that eventually, every kid will do this thinking, but it's good to get them to make a conscious effort to learn as they tinker... What you want is for kids to become conscious of how they are learning, what there is to learn, and what they know already. Once they've got this ability, there is no stopping their self-education."

Take note of that last term: *self-education*. It's an important step in the development of the self-leader, and it's never been easier to both develop and maintain than it is today. The learning process isn't done after 12 or 16 years—or more—when you take that certificate you've earned, frame it, hang it on your wall, and say "School's out!" It's not limited to the classroom or the lab. School's never out! All the world's knowledge and wisdom is—literally—right at your fingertips. So, to keep on leading, keep on learning. It's a trait that will serve you well—for a lifetime. As Michelangelo reportedly said at the age of 87, "Ancora Imparo" or, "yet, I am learning."

Explore the world. Nearly everything is really interesting if you go into it deeply enough. Work as hard and as much as you want to on the things you like to do the best.

~ Richard Feynman

A KINDRED SPIRIT

What brought the subject of tinkering to my mind recently was a new book by syndicated columnist and best-selling author Michelle Malkin. It's titled *Who Built That*, but it was her subtitle that got my attention: *Awe-Inspiring Stories of American Tinkerpreneurs*.

I'd barely opened the book when I discovered that I'd found a kindred spirit. There it was, on the second page, right in the opening paragraphs of the Introduction. She writes: "I am a tinkerer-wannabe. Among my contrivances gone wrong:

- a modified Weber grill that exploded and nearly burned my eyebrows off,

- a soda-bottle submarine that sank like a concrete block in the bathtub, and

- a cache of defective marshmallow shooters clogged up with sticky-sweet ammunition."

A kindred spirit indeed! In an earlier book, *Ingredients of Outliers*, I wrote about some of my own entrepreneurial misadventures, including:

- The Shufeldt Wine Aerator,

- A vibrating tampon called the Vibrapon (intended to reduce menstrual cramps), and

- A company called *Dead TV*, to produce and air obituaries on the Internet and cable TV.

Regarding my tinkering flops, I wrote: "But I learned—and learning is the key. The point is this: if you approach failure as simply a hurdle to jump or an event from which you can learn, failing's not so bad."

Malkin had a similar response: "I'm proud of my discards. In failure, after all, lies progress. In misadventure lies enlightenment. Disappointment and dead ends induce turnarounds. Turnarounds yield new and endless paths toward improvement and success."

She continues: "I believe I am uniquely qualified to write a book celebrating unsung American inventors and entrepreneurs who've actually succeeded. Who better than an obsessive geek tinkerer-wannabe to tell the stories of these unappreciated geniuses and business phenoms?"

Given my own fondness for tinkering, I love the word she coined— Tinkerpreneurs. I wish I'd thought of it. She describes them as: "underappreciated inventors and innovators of mundane things who changed the world by successfully commercializing their ideas and creating products, companies, jobs, and untold opportunities that endure today... They were tireless, self-made, and largely self-taught."

"Self-taught," says Malkin, or, as Gabrielson put it, "self-educated." Hmmm! Perhaps they're on to something. Let's see.

BY VIRTUE OF EXPERIENCE

Born in a small community in Italy in 1870, there was nothing in Maria's early years to suggest the revolutionary impact she would later have on education systems and methods around the world. When she was three, her family moved to Rome where, fortunately, she would gain access to schools which would later feed her growing hunger to learn. Her father, a mid-level government official, had no interest in raising an educated daughter (an all-too-common attitude of 19th century dads), but Maria's well-educated mother provided the encouragement that would launch her career.

Maria did well in school, especially in the sciences and mathematics, and began planning for a career in engineering. Then, at age 20, she switched to medicine and, upon completing her studies several years later at the University of Rome, Maria Montessori became Italy's first female doctor.

In medical school, she had shown strong interest in pediatrics and psychiatry and began her career both in emergency medicine and pediatrics, working closely with children experiencing some degree of mental disability. Her reputation grew rapidly, both nationally and internationally, as an advocate of women's rights and the education of children with learning difficulties.

In 1900, Dr. Montessori was named co-director of a new school, launched to train teachers of mentally challenged children. During her two years there, she designed and developed methods and materials which she would later adapt for teaching children in mainstream education. Thus was born what would become the world-renowned Montessori Method. By the time of her death in 1952, at age 81, there were thousands of Montessori classrooms around the world.

Montessori was an outspoken critic of what was then considered the "normal and correct" way to teach children (and, sadly, still is in many places). She wrote: "If education is always to be conceived along the same antiquated lines of a mere transmission of knowledge, there is little to be hoped from it in the bettering of man's future." On another occasion, she described the world of education as "like an island where people, cut off from the world, are prepared for life by exclusion from it."

In explaining the Montessori Method, she wrote; "We discovered that education is not something which the teacher does, but that it is a natural process which develops spontaneously in the human being. It is not acquired by listening to words, but in virtue of experiences in which the child acts on his environment."

My kids are Montessori graduates. Both attended a Montessori school from preschool through eighth grade, and I witnessed firsthand the effect of the "Montessori way." To this day, many years later, I can still see the Montessori way shine in their actions and traits. They're respectful, confident, inquisitive, and always learning.

I will not follow where the path may lead, but I will go where there is no path, and I will leave a trail.

~ Muriel Strode

ALIVE AND WELL

It's been some 65 years since the trailblazing Maria Montessori passed on, but her legacy is alive and well. In one of our recent books, *Outliers in Education*, we profiled a woman named Mary Vallelonga, who has been teaching for about 40 years, most of them dedicated to the Montessori Method.

In an interview, we asked Vallelonga what it is that sets a Montessori classroom apart from a traditional one. "Everything's different," she said, "from the beautiful materials, to learning at your own pace, to not being judged, to the non-competitive classroom situation, to not being graded, and being in a multi-aged classroom, where the younger ones are learning from the older ones, and the older ones are feeling like mentors and leaders. That's Montessori!

"In a traditional classroom, you have a teacher standing before his or her students teaching a certain curriculum. They're the focal point. The eyes are upon the teacher because the teacher has something important to say. In a Montessori classroom, as Maria Montessori said, 'We must become invisible.'"

Asked what advice she might offer to those who want their learning to continue outside the classroom walls, Vallelonga replied: "One of the most important things you can do is to find people in your life who can be mentors for you. I've had wonderful mentors throughout my life, who thought what I had to say was worthy of hearing."

MENTORING: A DUAL ROLE

Mary Vallelonga's advice about the important role mentors can play in your life is spot on. That's something I missed out on during my adolescent years. I wasn't fortunate enough to be introduced to a mentor—someone who would have opened doors, kicked me in the rear end, or patted me on the back, as necessary. I take complete responsibility for this. I simply didn't put myself out there to investigate the possibilities of what a mentor could do to help me. Consequently, I was my own best and worst counsel and, subsequently, I made lots of mistakes along the way. Persevering through these mistakes, and reading books, as well as watching others, became my pseudo-mentor.

By the time I got to medical school, I'd become keenly aware of the importance of mentoring. I promised myself I'd mentor anyone who asked (and some who didn't) in whatever ways I could, to offer up any knowledge or, at the very least, tell them all the ways I screwed up.

FLIPPING THE SWITCH

Kelli was a junior in high school who wanted to become a doctor. I was introduced to her by our marketing director, who was very active in a great organization called Young Life, where she mentored Kelli. Once I got to know her, Kelli told me she'd been headed down the wrong path with a group of friends influencing negative choices, and made a conscious effort to change her peer group. This is when she flipped the switch to creating the kind of future she really wanted.

Kelli was, in a word, fearless. She learned to fly at 16, did well in school, and was accepted to a private college where she continued to excel. While on breaks, she'd shadow me in the emergency department and soak up anything she could. She went on to graduate from college, got married, and got accepted to medical school. She and I wrote a number of articles together, and we stay in touch to this day.

One of my proudest memories was watching her walk across the stage during her graduation. Today, she's a plastic surgery resident in a prestigious East Coast medical center. It gives me great satisfaction to know Kelli will go on, in her humble yet fearless way, to care for her patients, change the world, and impact and mentor a whole new generation of doctors who, in turn, pay it forward to the next group of aspiring physicians.

As a teenager, Kelli was wiser than I was, in that she sought out guidance. That's the thing to do. Don't just sit back and wait for a mentor to show up on your doorstep. Tell everyone you know that you want to interview someone who has your dream job. If they don't know someone who matches what you're looking for, chances are they might know someone else who does. If networking doesn't turn up much, start googling professionals in your area. If you don't know your dream job title, check out the field you're interested in. See what comes up.

After doing some research on your potential mentor, it's time to reach out. Email or call this potential mentor, and introduce yourself. Explain why you're contacting him or her. Ask for advice. A simple request, saying "I want to become a [that person's profession], and would love to ask you a few questions," could be the beginning of an incredible mentorship experience.

Most young people would probably be too intimidated to do that, no matter how much they wish they could. But self-leaders realize the worst they can get is a "No," so they keep going until they find mentors for themselves.

Mentoring is a way to pass on what you know, and it works both ways—finding someone who can teach you the ropes and then showing the ropes to someone else.

~ Brandon Johnson

For me, mentoring harkens back to an earlier era. It's been some three hundred years since famed English scientist Sir Isaac Newton wrote, in a letter to a colleague, "If I have seen farther it is by standing on the shoulders of giants." I would echo those words today. If, for a few people, I can be a metaphorical "giant" so others can see and go farther, then at least in my mind, I've left the world a better place than when I entered it, which is as much as anyone can hope for.

CONCLUSION

I dare you: commit to exploring the "whys" that pop into your head. I've built a life by questioning the world, and I couldn't be happier or more grateful. The answers to the questions you raise might lead you to some surprising findings: about yourself, the way you view the world, the way things work, the way life works. Constant learning is the way to a life full of wonder, and a life of continual growth. I can say with true conviction that my commitment to learn all I can from my experiences has made me who I am today.

—————— TAKEAWAYS ——————

- **Enroll** in a course. For example, Udemy (www.udemy.com) and Coursera (www.coursera.org) offer great, free courses on a broad range of topics.

- **Ask questions** that begin with "how" and "why." They'll yield much richer responses. Accept the answers, then verify them.

- **Watch** a TED talk on a subject you don't know much about.

- **Keep an open mind.** Approaching situations, conversations, and new people with an open mind, you're likely to learn a great deal.

- **Change** what you do for physical exercise. Learn to box, mountain bike, golf, row, or salsa. Your brain learns when your body learns.

- **Learn more about yourself,** too. Introspection is your best friend. Learn to question yourself, and to accept the answers you find.

- **Put down the remote.** Learn a new card game, and unwind in a way that challenges your mind.

- **Make "why" one of your favorite words.** There's a reason three-year-olds love this word. They're dying to learn about the world, and the way it works. Rediscover that same curiosity within yourself. Allow yourself to ask "why," even when it may seem silly.

- **Rethink your definition of curiosity.** Far too often, people think curiosity is just aimless mental wandering. When you allow your mind to wander—and wonder, you'll find treasures, many of which can be lucrative.

5

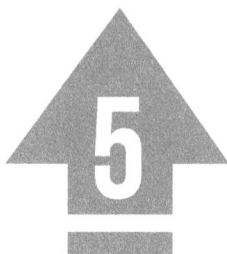

PERSISTENCE: FROM STUMBLING BLOCKS TO STEPPING STONES

Nothing in the world can take the place of persistence.
Talent will not; nothing is more common that unsuccessful men
with talent. Genius will not; unrewarded genius is almost a Proverb.
Education will not; the world is full of educated failures.
Persistence and determination alone are omnipotent.

~ Calvin Coolidge

The above words, spoken nearly a century ago by the 30th President of the United States, have long been favorites of mine. They epitomize a core principle on which our nation was founded, and on which it has been shaped. Call it what you will—persistence, determination, resolve, tenacity, perseverance, steadfastness—it's the quality of pressing on toward a goal, no matter what obstacles or difficulties may stand in the way.

I've encountered a variety of obstacles during my journey through life and have done my best to climb them, push through them, or work around them. I chose to view them, not as stumbling blocks, but as stepping stones. For example, in 1993, I started a company called NextCare Urgent Care—what would eventually become a group of walk-in clinics—on a shoestring, and with the help of a small bank loan. I literally worked day and night to get it up and running. During its early stage, one partner backed out and another one said he didn't want to take on any more risk but stuck in there for the crazy ride.

I pressed on, and we were actually making headway when our banker informed us our loan was being transferred to the "workout" division. At the time, I thought this was great, because I liked to work out. Then I learned that this division was where bad loans were handled. The bank could have called the note at any time, which meant it would have taken over and seized all our assets.

So my wife and I triple mortgaged our home and I finally switched banks. When I went back and asked our "workout banker" why he hadn't simply demanded payment, he told me it was because he never heard defeat in my voice. I served as chairman and CEO of NextCare until 2010, by which time it had grown from a single clinic to fifty-eight clinics in six states, with annualized revenue of nearly one hundred million dollars.

Now maybe I'm just too dumb to quit, but remember: You're never beaten till you quit. For those who get into fights, the worst people to fight with are those who never quit, because they just keep coming back for more.

Here's the bottom line: if it was easy, everyone would do it. With ordinary talent and extraordinary perseverance, all things are attainable.

THE LAST LECTURE

A number of years ago, while he was dying of pancreatic cancer (a fierce and aggressive form of cancer), Professor Randy Pausch gave an inspirational lecture on life and attaining childhood dreams. It was part of a series hosted by Carnegie Mellon University where professors were asked to think about what they'd want the world to know if they could only give one "last lecture." Pausch was invited after his cancer came back a second time, and he was given mere months to live. The word "last" rang a little truer in his situation.

The lecture, where he talked about achieving childhood dreams, was recorded, uploaded online, and has been viewed on YouTube more than seventeen million times. From working for Disney as an Imagineer, to experiencing zero gravity, to creating virtual realities, Pausch worked tirelessly to see many of his childhood dreams come to fruition. In addressing the topic of obstacles, or "brick walls" as he called them, Pausch wisely insists that, "the brick walls are there for a reason. The brick walls are not there to keep us out. The brick walls are there to give us a chance to show how badly we want something. Because the brick walls are there to stop the people who don't want it badly enough. They're there to stop the other people."

I've come to relish the challenging opportunities. The higher the bar, the more difficult the challenge for everyone else as well. Though, it wasn't always this way for me. As a seventh-grader, I quit the eighth-grade football team after getting my butt kicked for ten days during "two-a-days." I hated how that made me feel and decided I'd never let it happen again.

There have been many times in my life when quitting would have been the easier and sometimes even the smarter thing to do. Yet, every time the thought crossed my mind, I'd have a flashback to seventh grade and double down on my resolve. Thus, I've turned into one of those people who'll fight to the last drop of blood.

Mind you, I've never been to the last drop of blood, so that's easy for me to say. I do, however, read books about men and women who've had their backs against the wall and managed not only to survive their trials but overcome them and ultimately "knock it out of the park."

Be like a postage stamp—stick to one
thing until you get there.
~ Margaret Carty

Perseverance, determination, tenacity, persistence — or whatever term you choose — is the "secret sauce" which separates the achievers from the wishful thinkers. Let me share a few of their stories with you.

THE WILD BLUE YONDER

As a child, Cecilia Aragon was so afraid of heights that merely climbing a ladder caused her to break out in a sweat. Even the simple act of shaking hands with someone terrified her. To overcome her fears, she said: "I realized that if I was ever going to do anything, I had to expand my comfort zone pretty dramatically." Today, she's an award-winning computer scientist and university professor.

But there's a lot more to her story. As a graduate student, she swallowed her fear of heights and accepted an invitation from a friend to take a flight in a small, four-seater airplane. During the flight, her friend challenged her to take the controls. Impulsively, she agreed. It proved to be a life-changing experience. "When I was growing up," she said, "my big dilemma was whether to become a scientist or an artist. Becoming a pilot was absolutely the furthest thing from my mind."

As soon as the plane landed, Aragon signed up for flying lessons. "I was in heaven," she recalled. "This is my dream. This is it." But turning one's dreams into reality can be hard. Lacking the financial resources she needed for her lessons, she had to take on two jobs, often working eighty to one hundred hours a week and squeezing what little time she had left into flying. But she was determined. She kept telling herself that "where there's a dream, there's a way," and she made it happen.

So long as there is breath in me, that long will I persist.
For now I know one of the greatest principles of success:
if I persist long enough I will win.

~ Og Mandino

In 1991, six years after her first solo flight, she was invited to join the United States Aerobatic Team. She still holds the record for the shortest time to do so, and was also the first Latina to win a spot on the team. During her four years on the team, her skills as a daredevil pilot helped her amass dozens of trophies. Today she's among the world's leading aerobatic pilots, and I assume she's no longer afraid of climbing a ladder.

Today, in addition to an active schedule in the air, Aragon continues her distinguished career as a computer scientist. She earned a B.S. degree in mathematics at the California Institute of Technology and a Ph.D. in computer science at the University of California, Berkeley. She's an Associate Professor at the University of Washington, and the director of its Human-Centered Data Science Lab. As a researcher, she has shown the same determination in the lab as she has in the air. In 2009, in recognition of her work, she received the prestigious Presidential Early Career Award for Scientists and Engineers.

AN UNLIKELY BALLERINA

Misty Copeland was thirteen years old when she first sought admission to a ballet school. In abruptly rejecting her application, school officials told the young African-American girl she had "the wrong body for ballet and was too old to be considered."

Well—unkindness aside—in the world of ballet, where budding ballerinas begin their training at age five, being considered too old at thirteen is understandable. Besides, Copeland had shown little interest in ballet. Much of her early life had been spent in poverty, living in a rundown motel in a Los Angeles suburb with her mother and five siblings. She'd never seen a ballet nor had she ever heard any classical music.

At age seven, she had seen a video of famed gymnast Nadia Comaneci, who won three gold medals in the 1976 Olympic Games and two more in 1980. What captivated Copeland was what she would later describe as "the joy of movement." Her mother had studied dance and had been a cheerleader for the National Football League's Kansas City Chiefs, and Copeland's older sister had been a standout on the Dana Middle School drill team. Not surprisingly, when Copeland arrived on the scene, she soon caught the attention of its drill team coach, Elizabeth Cantine. And Copeland later became the team captain.

After school, Copeland began going to the local Boys & Girls Club where Cantine's friend Cynthia Bradley, a former professional dancer, taught a free weekly ballet class. Bradley noticed Copeland's talent and potential, and became her mentor and ballet teacher. Copeland quickly closed the gap between herself and the ballerinas eight years ahead of her. For example, it normally takes a beginner about two years to learn to dance *en pointe* (on the tips of the toes); it took Copeland a mere three months. And, by age fifteen, she'd begun earning awards.

The next few years were hard for Copeland. For a time, she lived with the Bradley family, until her mother, Sylvia DelaCerna demanded that she return home and give up dancing. DelaCerna believed the Bradleys had exerted too much influence on her daughter, and the situation quickly escalated to a well-publicized custody battle, including an emancipation filing and various restraining orders. For Copeland, it became what she later described as "a nomadic existence," and a painful one. Eventually, all claims and counterclaims were withdrawn and Copeland was able to continue her rise to ballet stardom.

But some obstacles remained. In 2012, nearing the pinnacle of her career, she began experiencing severe pain in her left leg. By fall, it had become intense and she was diagnosed with a half-dozen stress fractures of her *tibia*. Doctors warned her she might never dance again, but her surgery was successful and, after a few months of rest, she returned to the stage.

Walk that walk and go forward all the time.
Don't just talk that talk, walk it and go forward.
~ Chris Gardner

For many years, Copeland has been a part of the American Ballet Theatre (ABT), one of the premier classical ballet companies in the country. She joined ABT in 2000 as a member of its Corps de Ballet. In August 2007, she was named a soloist, one of the youngest ballerinas to reach that level. She continued to excel, and was soon assigned leading roles in various productions. She has performed numerous times at New York's famed Metropolitan Opera House, and for audiences across the U.S. and around the world, including Beijing, London, and Brisbane. On June 30, 2015, she reached the pinnacle of her ballet career, when the ABT promoted her to its highest level, principal dancer. She is the first African-American woman to earn that position in the 75-year history of the ABT.

Misty Copeland's achievements have by no means been limited to her skills as a ballerina, as spectacular as those skills are. In May 2015, she was named to *TIME* magazine's 100 Most Influential People in the World. That same month, she was featured in a segment on the CBS program *60 Minutes* and, more recently, performed on *The Late Show with Stephen Colbert*, accompanied by world-famous cellist Yo-Yo Ma.

In 2014, President Barack Obama appointed her to the President's Council on Fitness, Sports & Nutrition, and she has become a highly visible advocate of increased opportunities for minorities and the underprivileged in the world of ballet. Young African-Americans now make up a significant portion of her audiences. She told one interviewer: "For young African-Americans to feel that they have a chance to see a brown face on the stage, that ballet isn't this white world that's untouchable to them—I think having that visual does so much," she says. "I think it's so important for them to see me and to hear me."

Copeland has also written two books, both published in 2014. *Firebird* is an illustrated picture book for aspiring ballerinas, while *Life in Motion: An Unlikely Ballerina* has been a best-seller, about her own unlikely and amazing life story.

So, what's been the "secret sauce" that has propelled this once poor child from obscurity to the ranks of the world's most influential people—in less than 25 years? She's quick to mention "hard work and perseverance. You can do anything you want, even if you're being told negative things. Stay strong and find motivation."

THE VOICE OF A CHILD

Virtually everyone who aspires to become a self-leader recognizes the importance of education, but few have taken it to the level of a young Pakistani girl named Malala Yousafzai. Raised under an oppressive Taliban regime that not only discouraged the education of females but even blocked them from attending school, Yousafzai decided to speak out and make a change.

Born in Pakistan in 1997, her passion for education began early. Her family operated a chain of schools and encouraged her to not only a life of learning, but to become a spokesperson for the cause of female education. When the British Broadcasting Corporation (BBC) began seeking a local schoolgirl to blog anonymously about life under Taliban rule, no one stepped forward, so Yousafzai's father, Ziauddin Yousafzai, volunteered her for the role. In an effort to conceal her identity, she used a pseudonym for her blog entries.

It was a dangerous time to espouse such a cause. The Taliban had not only issued an order banning girls from attending school, but had been blowing up girls' schools in her hometown. But Malala Yousafzai would not be silenced. Shortly after starting her blog, her father took her to speak to a group of journalists in the larger city of Peshawar. In her speech, which was widely covered by the media, she demanded: "How dare the Taliban take away my basic right to education?" At the time, she was eleven years old!

The BBC blog was shut down a year later, and Yousafzai and her father were approached by a *New York Times* reporter about filming a documentary spelling out her passion for female education. More and more people rallied to her cause, and she began speaking regularly on television about its importance.

To make our way, we must have firm resolve,
persistence, tenacity. We must gear ourselves to
work hard all the way. We can never let up.

~ Ralph Bunche

Her fame grew and, in 2011, Archbishop Desmond Tutu, the well-known and respected activist from South Africa, nominated her for the International Children's Peace Prize. Shortly thereafter, the Pakistani government awarded her its first National Youth Peace Prize, followed by its National Peace Award for Youth. At age fourteen, Yousafzai's passion for education had brought her international recognition and influence.

But Taliban leaders had no intention of standing idly by as this child, this schoolgirl, dared to continue stirring up opposition to their rule. They decided she had to be silenced. On October 9, 2012, as Yousafzai was homeward bound on a bus, a gunman boarded it and shot her in the head. The bullet traveled through her head and her neck, before becoming embedded in her shoulder.

The news of her shooting brought outcries from around the world, as the medical community rushed to her aid. After emergency treatment at local hospitals, she was flown to Great Britain where she was treated at the Queen Elizabeth Hospital in Birmingham, which specializes in caring for military personnel wounded in battle. Yousafzai would go on to recover completely, with her resolve to continue her fight stronger than ever.

On July 12, 2013, her sixteenth birthday and less than a year after her shooting, Yousafzai spoke at the United Nations. In her speech, she said: "The terrorists thought they would change my aims and stop my ambitions, but nothing changed in my life except this: weakness, fear and hopelessness died. Strength, power and courage was born... I'm here to speak up for the right of education for every child. I want education for the sons and daughters of the Taliban and all terrorists and extremists."

Her book, *I Am Malala: The Story of the Girl Who Stood Up for Education and Was Shot by the Taliban*, was published in October 2013. Reviewers called it "riveting" and "fearless," and one likened it to *The Diary of Anne Frank*. In October 2014, Yousafzai received the Nobel Peace Prize for her work. At age seventeen, she was the youngest person to ever receive that award. On her eighteenth birthday, July 12, 2015, she opened a school in Lebanon for Syrian refugee girls from the ages of fourteen to eighteen.

In her book, she wrote: "Let us remember: One book, one pen, one child and one teacher can change the world." As one who has clearly shown her ability as a self-leader since she was a young girl, Malala Yousafzai remains determined to change the world, even risking her life for the cause.

If you push through the resistance and keep driving for what you want, you will ultimately achieve rewards beyond any you had hoped for.

~ T. Boone Pickens

CHANGING COURSE

In one of our recent books, *Outliers in Law*, we interviewed a young professional named David Medina, a recent graduate of the Sandra Day O'Connor College of Law at Arizona State University. He is currently serving as a law clerk for a U.S. District Court judge. But until a few years ago, becoming a lawyer wasn't even on his radar. Throughout high school, Medina had visualized a career in engineering, math or science. A good student, he graduated from high school ranked third in a class of 750.

Medina enrolled at Stanford University, expecting similar success. "In my mind, I could do no wrong," he said, "but when I arrived at

Stanford, it was an entirely different ballgame." He did earn his bachelor's degree but, by his own admission, he put very little effort into it, and had no idea what he'd do next. After marking time for a couple of years, he decided to go to law school.

"I crushed law school," he reports. "After feeling bad about my undergraduate performance, I was determined to commit as much time and energy as I needed to excel. That's when I flipped the switch."

Asked to explain what he meant, he said: "Flipping the switch is when self-leadership kicks in. It means deciding you're going to change and give it everything you've got. Flipping the switch means you're going to be the one to say, 'You know what? My future begins with me.'" I asked him if we could steal that line for this book, I liked it so much!

Make a choice. You have the ability to have an amazing life, but you have to be the one to flip the switch.

CONCLUSION

The leaders in this book are incredibly high achievers, but they're also normal people. What they share is their refusal to give up on their dreams, and to never be a victim. Instead, they took control, and scaled the proverbial brick walls.

They're no different than you, save for being pushed far enough and long enough to dig their heels in and succeed. You can too!

─────────── **TAKEAWAYS** ───────────

- **Place yourself** in uncomfortable situations and work through the challenge. This could simply mean running through pain, speaking to a group when you feel like throwing up from anxiety, or sticking with a friend who's draining your capacity.

- **Welcome challenges.** They make life interesting and, once accomplished, fuel a feeling of pride and accomplishment. If it was easy, everyone would do it. It's the hard stuff that makes it fun!

- **Continue to strive** for success. If you're persistent, you'll get it. If you're consistent, you'll keep it. If you ultimately fail, you'll learn.

- **Redefine success.** Know that success never comes without challenges.

- **Bring a rain jacket.** Be prepared to weather the storm. Yes, there will be storms. They're inevitable. It's how you deal with them that really matters.

- **Evaluate** whether or not the goals you've set for yourself align with your long-range plans. If not, rethink and rewrite them. Staying the course isn't easily done without clearly defined, specific, purposeful goals.

- **Get over it.** Sometimes, bad stuff happens. And sometimes, there's nothing you can do about it other than learn from it, and move on. Don't waste your time lamenting or fixating on something you need to let go. Let it go!

- **Just do it.** Work on the toughest things first. Successful people do the things unsuccessful people don't want to do. If you're having a difficult time with a project, split it into smaller pieces and tackle it one piece at a time.

6

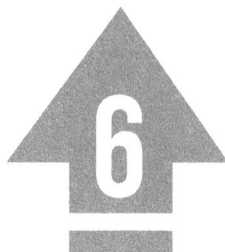

KINDNESS: IT CAN BE CONTAGIOUS

A single act of kindness throws out roots in all directions, and the roots spring up and make new trees. The greatest work that kindness does to others is that it makes them kind themselves.

~ Amelia Earhart

We all come from different backgrounds and have faced varying degrees of problems and opportunities in our lives. But one thing we all have in common—we've traveled a hard road at times. When things get tough, it feels good when we're treated warmly and with compassion. Kind words—encouraging words—can go a long way in helping us get over those inevitable bumps in the road.

I love the way Patrick Morley, best-selling author of *The Man in the Mirror* and many other books, expressed it: "Encouragement is food for the heart, and every heart is a hungry heart." Kind words not only ease the hunger in the hurting heart, but they work wonders in our own hearts as well. Life is so much easier when we treat others with the respect, kindness, and compassion they deserve. It's even more fun when they don't expect that compassion. It feels great to see people "light up" when you treat them with kindness.

Ken Blanchard, business leader and best-selling author of *The One Minute Manager*, has long advocated the importance of treating team members with kindness. He was an early advocate of the principle of "management by walking around," the purpose of which is to spot employees doing things right, rather than doing them wrong. "People who feel good about themselves produce good results," he said, "and people who produce good results feel good about themselves."

Self-leaders demonstrate kindness when they treat everyone within their sphere of influence in the same way, regardless of position or rank or relationship. It doesn't matter if they're talking with the top-ranking executives or the newest trainee, they never "pull rank," but treat everyone with kindness and respect. In doing so, they earn the respect of those they lead.

Kindness is the kingpin of success in life; it is the prime factor in overcoming friction and making the human machinery run smoothly.

~ Andrew Chapman

A CHILD'S INNOCENCE

When my daughter Kaleigh was six years old, she started talking to me about another child in her first-grade class. No matter how hard she tried, she couldn't describe him in enough detail for me to figure out which classmate she was talking about. She finally said, "Daddy, you know his father, he owns a restaurant."

I finally realized she was talking about an African-American boy in her class, whose father owned a chain of barbeque restaurants. I'll never forget the fact that it didn't even occur to her to mention the color of his skin. She was race indifferent and remains so to this day. I couldn't be prouder of her for seeing the person and not the color of his skin.

Kindness is more than deeds. It is an
attitude, an expression, a look, a touch. It
is anything that lifts another person.
~ C. Neil Strait

Lovingkindness, whether it comes naturally or is something you have to work on, may be the most important trait of all for the self-leader. Leaders don't evaluate others based on their race, color, appearance, religion, politics, sexual orientation, gender identity, or other factors. As an emergency room physician, I regularly encounter patients in every kind of distress—drunk, dirty, bleeding, and belligerent. But, as my daughter taught me, I strive to see each of my patients as simply human and treat all those who come through our emergency department doors with lovingkindness and compassion, regardless of what condition they may be in.

Last year, around the holidays, a certain patient had just been released from our emergency department. After discharge, he turned right around and checked in again. This time, I was the one who treated him. I asked him what was wrong and he said it was the exact same thing for which he'd just been treated and released. So I said, "I understand you have this issue, but what do you really need?" He replied, "I need $130 for a bus ticket to Oakland so I can collect my inheritance from my father, who died a month ago."

I knew he probably wasn't telling me the truth. However, I gave him $150 and said, "Buy yourself some food for the bus ride and best of luck to you!" Then, I had one of our security people drive him to the bus station. About 10 days later, he showed up again in our ED. The nurse who'd assisted on his earlier visit was on duty again and called him on it and shamed him into leaving.

When she told me the story, I have to admit I laughed. If that $150 helped him even a little bit to get on his feet, then it was all good. It wasn't the first time I fell for a sob story and it won't be the last. I'd rather fall for them a hundred times for the chance of helping one person, rather than turning a blind eye on everyone.

One final caveat on kindness that may be the most important point: the lovingkindness has to extend to yourself as well.

"IT'S YOUR LUCKY DAY!"

One wintry day in February 2014, young Myles Eckert and his family were on their way to lunch at a local restaurant. Snow had fallen the night before, and there was still plenty of it on the ground as they carefully made their way across the parking lot. Then something lying in the snow caught Myles' eye. Reaching down, he saw it was a $20 bill, and quickly retrieved it, as visions of the video game he'd buy danced in his head.

Then, as the family entered the restaurant, Myles caught a glimpse of something—or rather someone—that immediately erased any thoughts of video games. Suddenly, he knew exactly what he was going to do with that $20 bill. As soon as he spotted a man sitting at one of the restaurant tables, a whole new plan began taking shape in his mind.

If we all do one random act of kindness daily, we just might set the world in the right direction.
~ Martin Kornfeld

The man he saw was wearing a military uniform. His name: Lt. Col. Frank Dailey, a member of the Ohio National Guard. Myles quickly scrawled a note, which read: "Dear soldier, My Dad was a soldier. He's in heaven now. I found this $20 in the parking lot when we got here. We like to pay it forward in my family. It's your lucky day! Thank you for your service."

Myles never had a chance to meet his dad. Army Sergeant Andy Eckert was killed in Iraq in 2005, just a few weeks after Myles was born. But the boy visits the gravesite often to keep his Dad "in the know."

Colonel Dailey was deeply moved by Myles' kindness. After sharing the story with his wife, they decided to tell other family members about it by posting it on their Facebook page. What happened next could be described in Amelia Earhart's words: "a single act of kindness throwing out roots in all directions." His story went viral.

When Steve Hartman of CBS News heard the story, he arranged to meet with Myles and share the story on his popular "On the Road" segment of the CBS Evening News. Before long, it had been seen more than a half-million times. Other media outlets picked up the story, and many total strangers began offering cash and other gifts to Myles and his family. Instead, they decided to point donors in the direction of an organization called Snowball Express, which arranges free vacations for boys and girls who have lost a military parent in the line of duty. So the roots of Myles' kindness continue "to spring up and make new trees."

When I first heard this touching story, I was surprised at how many of the qualities of the self-leader Myles displayed, in addition to his loving-kindness. They included humility, integrity, maturity, generosity, and initiative. The reason for my surprise: when he wrote that note and gave Colonel Dailey the money, he was merely eight years old!

INTO THE WILD BLUE YONDER

Let me tell you about Amelia Earhart, whose thoughts on the importance of kindness introduced this chapter. Her name is probably familiar to you, even if you don't know her story. It's been nearly 80 years since she disappeared—literally—from the face of the earth. A self-leader in every respect, she had determined, from an early age, to make her own way. Born in Kansas in 1897, she was a pioneer in the early days of aviation. She got her first plane ride when she was 23. It lasted 10 minutes, but it would change her life. "By the time I had got two or three hundred feet off the ground," she commented, "I knew I had to fly." And fly she did!

Earhart began a series of jobs in order to acquire the $1,000 she needed for flying lessons. To reach the airfield where the lessons were given meant a long bus ride, followed by a four-mile walk. But she persisted and, in 1923, she became the sixteenth woman ever to be granted a pilot's license. She'd go on to set records: among others, the first woman to fly solo across the North American continent and back; and the first woman to fly solo across the Atlantic Ocean.

These were spectacular accomplishments in those early days of aviation, and made Earhart world famous. Congress awarded her the Distinguished Flying Cross, President Herbert Hoover presented her with the National Geographic Society's Gold Medal, and the French government bestowed on her one of its most prestigious awards.

Earhart also enjoyed competing in air races, including the first Women's Air Derby, from Santa Monica to Cleveland, an event humorist Will Rogers dubbed "The Powder-Puff Derby." The race included several intermediate stops. At one of the final ones, she learned she was tied for the lead with a friend named Ruth Nichols. For the final leg, Nichols was to take off first but, as she neared the end of the runway, her plane struck a tractor and flipped over.

Rather than taking off, with victory all but assured, Earhart ran to her friend and pulled her from the plane. It wasn't until she made sure Nichols wasn't injured that she took off. Instead of winning, she finished third, but what she had done symbolized the courage and selflessness she demonstrated so often.

Earhart's passion for aviation was by no means limited to her time in the air. In fact, her efforts in promoting the young aviation industry had far greater impact than any of her individual accomplishments. For example, she was a founder and the first president of "the Ninety-Nines," an organization of women pilots dedicated to mutual support and advocacy. She spoke and wrote often on behalf of aviation in general and women's roles in it. Her goal, she once said, was to make America "air-minded," and to show that flying was no longer just for "daredevils and supermen."

You cannot get through a single day without having an impact on the world around you. What you do makes a difference, and you have to decide what kind of difference you want to make.

~ Jane Goodall

How much of an impact did her efforts have? Well, even though she was missing and presumed dead by the time World War II began, she has been credited with inspiring a generation of women pilots, including the more than one thousand members of the Women Airforce Service Pilots (WASP). During the war, they logged more than sixty million miles ferrying military aircraft, towing gliders and targets, and freeing their male counterparts for combat missions.

Earlier, on July 2, 1937, Earhart had disappeared, somewhere over the South Pacific. She and her navigator, Fred Newman, had completed about 22,000 miles of their planned 29,000-mile flight around the world. As they were nearing a small island which was to be their next stop, radio contact was lost. Search efforts began immediately and today, amazingly, they continue. The most common theory is that they ran out of fuel, crashed at sea, and perished. Nearly 80 years later, the search goes on, perhaps futilely, but may one day bring closure to the remarkable life of a woman who, in all she undertook, demonstrated what makes a self-leader tick.

CHANGING COURSE

To close the loop on this chapter, here's a glimpse into the life of a doctor I interviewed for the book, *Outliers in Medicine*. Her name is Robin Blackstone who, after graduating from medical school, fulfilled her internship and residency requirements, and began her practice as a general surgeon. In 1996, she established an Advanced Laparoscopic General Surgery and Surgical Oncology private practice in Scottsdale, Arizona. A bright future beckoned.

There was never any heart truly great and gracious
that was not also tender and compassionate.

~ Robert South

Then, in 2000, the picture changed. In a recent interview, she told us: "My practice was primarily centered in surgical oncology. I also did very advanced general surgery procedures with the laparoscope. During an especially stressful time, I became overwhelmed by emotion and felt I needed to take a serious break and think about the kind of medicine I was practicing. I closed my practice in September and took the next nine months off."

During that time, a local bariatric surgeon asked Dr. Blackstone to help him learn how to perform gastric bypass surgery laparoscopically. The request would change her life, and the lives of thousands of others who would become her patients. "After a few cases," she said, "I was really intrigued by this new specialty that was emerging in treating obese patients."

In November 2001, she established the Scottsdale Bariatric Center, to put together a comprehensive treatment plan for people who suffer from obesity and its related medical problems. To date, with one assistant, she has operated on and treated more than 5,000 people suffering from morbid obesity.

Asked what caused her to take a different direction in what was already an established professional career, she replied: "That's where I found my stride, in a sense, because it was to help people against whom it's still okay to be prejudiced and treated with disrespect—I hated that! They couldn't get access to the procedures that could help fix a lot of the medical problems they had. They were invisible to the medical profession, who had little scientific background to understand the truth about obesity, and didn't know how to help them. It totally captured my imagination and ignited within me a drive to help."

Blackstone's passion was reignited by the ability to serve with kindness a group that has been somewhat ignored by the medical community. When we practice kindness, kindness changes us.

SELF-LISTENING

In his book, *Let Your Life Speak: Listening for the Voice of Vocation*, author and teacher Parker J. Palmer describes how, years ago, he came across an old Quaker saying, which he would later use as the first four words of his book's title. He took them to mean: "Let the highest truths and values guide you. Live up to those demanding standards in everything you do." They meant following in the footsteps of such men and women as Dr. Martin Luther King, Jr., Mahatma Gandhi, Rosa Parks, or Mother Teresa, and others like them.

He described his efforts to emulate them as "rarely admirable, often laughable, and sometimes grotesque." He was, he said, trying to live a life that was other than his own.

Years later, he discovered an entirely new meaning in that Quaker saying. He writes: "Before you tell your life what you intend to do with it, listen for what it intends to do with you. Before you tell your life what truths and values you have decided to live up to, let your life tell you what truths you embody, what values you represent."

He adds: "Vocation does not come from willfulness. It comes from listening. I must listen to my life and try to understand what it is truly about—quite apart from what I would like it to be about—or my life will never represent anything real in the world, no matter how earnest my intentions."

In his 2005 commencement address at Stanford University, Steve Jobs echoed a similar theme. "You can't connect the dots looking forward," he said. "You can only connect them looking backwards."

CONCLUSION

Life is so much more rewarding and fulfilling when your first and only instinct is to be kind to others. Being kind isn't something that needs prodding or a logical analysis. It's simply treating everyone you meet, no matter their lot in life, with respect and compassion. The look on people's face when they're treated gently, particularly when they're not used to it, is priceless and amazing.

———————— TAKEAWAYS ————————

- **Look** at examples of people going out of their way to be kind or compassionate and try to emulate them. No one in history has ever been "too kind."

- **Practice empathy.** As Atticus Finch said in *To Kill a Mockingbird*, "You never really understand a person until you consider things from his point of view… until you climb into his skin and walk around in it."

- **Make eye contact** and smile at people you encounter each day with whom you wouldn't normally engage. If you consciously try to lift someone's spirit, you'll likely lift yours as well.

- **Show that you care.** Remember things people tell you. Ask how that concert was, how someone's ill mother is doing, or how their child's soccer game went.

- **Show gratitude** by writing a handwritten note for someone who's done something kind for you.

- **Give kudos.** When you receive good service at a restaurant, or someone's doing a great job at work, tell them, and let their supervisor know, too.

- **Give a compliment.** It can be uplifting for both giver and recipient. Making someone smile is such a fantastic feeling.

- **Don't neglect you.** The self-leader develops a positive self-image and takes care of himself or herself physically, mentally, and spiritually.

7

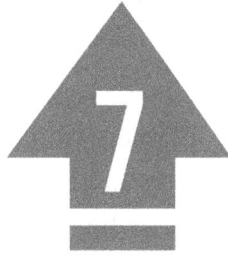

EQUANIMITY: KEEPING COOL'S A GOOD RULE

Great people are not affected by each puff of wind that blows ill. Like great ships, they sail serenely on, in a calm sea or a great tempest.
~ George Washington

Growing up, I was often on the receiving end of, probably, a well-deserved bout of screaming. Because I was a poor student, an average—at best—athlete and general goof-off, being yelled at was something with which I became quite familiar. Early on, I discovered an interesting thing about myself when people yelled at me; it had very little effect on me. I rarely remembered what they were yelling about or what I did wrong. However, I did remember the people "losing it" while they yelled. I remembered how contorted and red their faces became, and how embarrassed I felt for them for having so little control of their emotions.

As a resident assistant (R.A.) and hall director in college, it quickly became very clear to me that the students who stepped out of line responded much better when I had a non-confrontational, unemotional, but very direct conversation with them. Raising my voice had the opposite effect—they tuned me out. The one time I did yell at someone, and lifted him off his feet, was when a student fired a bottle rocket down the hall. He never did that again, but got "back at me" by marrying my former college girlfriend.

When I was an emergency medicine resident, I studied the communication style of Dr. Denise Fligner, who was one of my attending physicians. She talked very softly and slowly during the most life and death moments. Her style was at the opposite end of the spectrum from the other attending doctors, who would yell out orders and other comments. It was abundantly clear to me that the team, and sometimes even the patients, did much better under her calm and cool manner.

Through all those experiences, it is obvious that "losing your cool" never accomplishes the objective. It may, for a very short term, scare people into moving in a certain direction, but I've never seen it have any positive long-term effect.

All these years later, I still apply the lessons I learned from Dr. Fligner. When confronting critical, life and death situations, I know that having a calm, rational approach is much more likely to help the patient and the team. I've found that when I force myself to pause and take a deep breath, to slow down my speech and sharpen my senses, I think much more clearly.

Not long after receiving my pilot's license, my wife and I were flying across the country to a friend's wedding. We were flying VFR (Visual Flight Rules) at about 9,500 feet and quickly found ourselves in a rapidly worsening Midwest summer thunderstorm, which ultimately became a tornado. The air traffic controller with whom I was talking said in no uncertain terms (he was literally screaming at me over the radio) that our plane was surrounded by thunderstorms and to land immediately.

My wife René, who is as calm as I am, looked at me with wide eyes but said nothing. Fortunately, I was able to outwardly control my emotions, (inside, I was jumping out of my skin), pull the throttle back, lower the gear and circle down to an airport directly below. The moment we landed, all hell broke loose. The sky opened up, with high winds and large hail raining down on all the planes parked on the tarmac. We, literally, made it down with seconds to spare.

Without my previous experiences, I might have "lost it" and not been able to clearly think, or definitively act, in what was a life or death experience. In that storm, a minute of indecisive action or panic would have been fatal. I've been in four or five other intense, life or death experiences while flying, and countless times while treating critically ill patients in the emergency department. On every occasion, trying to be the calmest one in the room (even though I may be anxious on the inside) has always served me well.

Maybe you are the 'cool' generation. If coolness means a capacity to stay calm and use your head in the service of ends passionately believed in, then it has my admiration.

~ Kingman Brewster, Jr.

If you struggle with developing "Zen-like" equanimity when the going gets tough, how can you work on it? What works for me is to practice what pilots call "hangar flying," where they sit around in the hangar collectively brainstorming how to handle tough situations. I picture the worst thing that can happen, and how I'll react if it does. This way, I'm not surprised when the worst scenario does happen.

I do the same thing as an emergency physician. I'm regularly faced with treating patients with a wide range of life-threatening issues. To prepare, I rehearse the possible scenarios over and over again in my mind. What drugs will I need? What tools do I have? Who else is on the team? Finally, how do I deploy those resources to save the patient?

Doing a "hangar flight" saved my life a few years ago. One night, two pilot friends and I were discussing a flight we had planned for the next day, and we talked over some scenarios about what would happen if the plane crashed. The main issue with the plane we'd be flying was that it had only one door. If that door jams on impact due to a bent fuselage, the plane's occupants, if they survive the crash, often burn to death.

Nine hours after this discussion, the plane we were in did crash on takeoff and the airframe bent on impact when we struck a hangar. If my pilot friend in the rear seat hadn't kicked open the door before impact, we'd have burned to death, or died during the ensuing explosion. However, because we had considered our options and "hanger flew" the night before, we were able to remain calm and react decisively during that emergency.

> *One important key to success is self-confidence. An important key to self-confidence is preparation.*
> ~ Arthur Ashe

The key to equanimity is preparing for what could go wrong, in addition to the knowledge that losing your cool has the exact opposite effect of what you're hoping to accomplish, particularly in stressful situations.

THE LAST LECTURE

I can't imagine a greater tempest anyone can face than to be told in the prime of life that a terminal illness would soon bring premature death. Yet that was the tempest faced by a successful and popular young college professor, happily married with three small children, when told that a serious disease would soon claim his life.

I wrote a bit about him in Chapter 5. His name was Randolph Frederick "Randy" Pausch. Born in 1960, he was 46 when he was diagnosed with pancreatic cancer. A year later, he was told it was terminal and that he had three to six months to live. It was, of course, a cruel blow, but Pausch refused to spend even a moment feeling sorry for himself. His thoughts were for his family and how he could best prepare and equip them for life without him.

So he did something professors routinely do, he prepared a lecture. But there'd be nothing routine about this particular one. Designed for his wife Jai and their young children, it became known as "The Last Lecture." In it, he explained its purpose: "Somebody's going to push my family off a cliff pretty soon, and I won't be there to catch them. And that breaks my heart. But I have some time to sew some nets to cushion the fall. So, I can curl up in a ball and cry, or I can get to work on the nets."

Delivered in September 2007 at Carnegie Mellon University, where he taught computer science, it was later released on YouTube and, to date, has been re-shared and seen by millions around the world. Pausch later co-authored a book, also titled *The Last Lecture*, which quickly became a *New York Times* bestseller.

You have to try to take what life throws at you with grace and equanimity."
~ Christina Baker Kline

In the Introduction, he describes what he calls his "problem." It had nothing to do with his illness or impending death. Instead, he writes about how best to "teach my children what I would have taught them over the next twenty years." His solution was "The Last Lecture."

"I knew what I was doing that day," he explains, "I was trying to put myself in a bottle that would one day wash up on the beach for my children. If I were a painter, I would have painted for them. If I were a musician, I would have composed music. But I am a lecturer, so I lectured.

"I lectured about the joy of life, about how much I appreciated life, even with so little of my own left. I talked about honesty, integrity, gratitude, and other things I hold dear."

He spoke for more than an hour, without a trace of complaint or self-pity. He was calm and composed, and his message included lots of humor, much of it at his own expense. If you've never watched it, I highly recommend it. You'll find no sign of a dying man. Instead you'll see an example of equanimity at its absolute best, during the worst of times.

Today, nearly a decade after Randy Pausch's death, tributes continue to pour in, describing the life-changing impact of that message, initially heard by a few hundred, shared with millions, but aimed at an audience of just four.

BORN TO RUN

Unless you're into long-distance running—*really* long-distance running—chances are you've never heard of a young woman named Mira Rai. I hadn't either. Recently, though, my daughter Kaleigh brought her to my attention. It's quite a story, and I'd like to share it with you.

Rai is a native of Nepal, a small landlocked country in Asia, nestled primarily between India and China, and best known as the home of Mount Everest, the world's tallest mountain. Born in 1989, in a poverty-stricken village in the Himalayan mountain range, she lived in a mud hut without electricity or running water. Beginning at age eight, she spent her days, often from 4 a.m. to 7 p.m., running up and down steep and rough trails carrying heavy bags of rice and large buckets of water, in order to help provide for her family.

As so many others in that remote region did, Rai regularly ran those rugged mountain trails, though not for sport or exercise, but because they were often the only way to get from one place to another. Rai usually accompanied her mother on trips to the market, which was two days away. It was a lifestyle which helped her grow strong, confident and self-reliant. She would later say, "My parents were live-and-let-live, which gave me some opportunities."

Rai showed early signs of self-leadership. At the age of fourteen, she dropped out of school and spent two years in the Maoist army, in a noncombat role. When peace came, between the Maoist guerillas and the government, Rai was deemed a child combatant by the United Nations and was sent back home. When asked why she had joined the Maoist army at such a young age, she replied: "I was inspired by their message of making a better society here, especially for the women. While other girls were confined to their homes, I thought if I go out into the world, then others may follow."

We must choose each step we take with utmost caution, for the footprints we leave behind are as important as the path we will follow.

~ Lori R. Lopez

In 2014, when she first learned from friends that trail running was in fact a sport, Rai decided to try it out for herself, and entered a race in Kathmandu, Nepal's capital city. The friends had neglected to mention that it was a 50-kilometer (31+ mile) race, and Rai had never run even half that distance. She was the only woman to enter and, expecting perhaps a four-hour race, had brought neither food nor water with her. After running twice that long, she was fading quickly when a friend brought her some noodles and water. With that sustenance and help from her friend, Rai went on to finish the race in slightly more than nine hours.

Thus began a remarkable career. Rai quickly became an international celebrity. Within a little more than a year, she competed in 15 trail races, not only in Nepal, but in Hong Kong, Italy, Norway, France and Australia. And she won 12 of them.

In September 2015, Rai took on her biggest challenge, entering Spain's Ultra Pirineu, a 110-kilometer (68.35 mile) run that includes a climb of 22,000 feet. It was her longest and most difficult run by far. And, of the 75 women who entered, Rai finished second, a mere four minutes behind winner Emelie Forsberg, who is ranked among the top runners in the world. It was an incredible achievement and yet, in a post-race interview, she was calm and acted as if it were an everyday occurrence. When asked about the level of difficulty, Rai replied matter-of-factly: "Not difficult. For me, easy run. ... It was really fun, really good."

In an October 8, 2015 article headlined "Nepal's First Female Sports Star is a Trailblazing Global Hero," *Slate Magazine's* Sarah Barker wrote: "Rai has not only taken the trail running community by storm, she's become Nepal's first female sports star and a major celebrity in her country. Her head-spinning ascent over impossibly long odds goes beyond sports; it's the story of a pioneer, a precipitate of change, a social trailblazer."

When Barker, in an earlier interview, had asked Rai about the role attitude played in her life, she replied: "Relax, no hard work, just have fun... and not think about other things... I try not to think about anything other than keeping moving." When asked about the most difficult part of long-distance running, it was obvious that such a thought had never occurred to Rai. She simply laughed and described her long distance running as nothing more difficult than it being "comfortable."

By all accounts, Mira Rai remains the same person she's been all her life. Calmly and confidently, she continues to blaze a trail for the girls and women of Nepal, inspiring them to follow in her footsteps.

"NUTS!"

This is one of my favorite war stories. In the heat of battle, when the enemy has you seriously outnumbered and offers you the option of surrendering or being annihilated, maintaining your composure can be rather challenging, to say the least. Yet that's exactly the challenge U.S. Army Brigadier General Anthony C. McAuliffe faced during one of the most famous battles of World War II—best known as the Battle of the Bulge.

It was December 16, 1944 in Europe when German forces launched a major surprise attack against Allied troops. The latter had slowly but surely been recapturing European territory lost during the earlier days of the war and had just reached the strategic Rhine River. Desperate to stop them, Germany launched its attack with 200,000 men, a force that soon grew to 300,000, supported by more than a thousand tanks and 2,400 aircraft.

Confident of victory, the Germans sent a few men, under a truce flag, to present their demands to the commanding officer of the 101st Airborne Division, which was engaged in the defense of the Belgian city of Bastogne. As it turned out, the division was temporarily under the leadership of its deputy commanding officer, General McAuliffe.

The note offered "only one possibility to save the encircled U.S. troops from total annihilation: that is the honorable surrender of the encircled town." McAuliffe was given two hours to comply. If not, heavy artillery would immediately begin bombarding the town, endangering not only McAuliffe's troops but Bastogne's civilian population as well.

My father used to say to me, "Whenever you get into a jam, whenever you get into a crisis or an emergency, become the calmest person in the room and you'll be able to figure your way out of it."

~ Rudolph Giuliani

This was indeed the kind of "great tempest" George Washington had mentioned in the quote I used to introduce this chapter. Thousands of lives were at stake as well as the morale of the military and the people of the United States, and the clock was ticking. But there was no panic, no feeling of desperation. After calmly and briefly consulting with his officers, McAuliffe had a return note prepared. It contained only one word, one four-letter word of defiance, one word that would become legendary in the annals of American warfare. The note read simply: "Nuts!"

McAuliffe assigned Colonel Joseph Harper to deliver the note to the waiting German delegation. The German officer who read it seemed confused and asked what it meant. Harper replied without emotion: "In plain English, go to hell."

The German threat of artillery bombardment never materialized and, thanks to reinforcement by additional American troops, Bastogne was spared. For his role, General McAuliffe was later awarded both the Distinguished Service Cross and the Distinguished Service Medal. In 1949, the story of his calm defiance was told in the movie *Battleground*.

AN ENGLISH TEACHER

In *Outliers in Education*, part of the Outliers Series featuring inspirational men and women who excel in their chosen fields, I tell the story of Clark Sturges, a man who has worn many hats, including author, publisher, editor, and teacher. In that last-named role, he served as a professor of English for 38 years at Diablo Valley College in Pleasant Hill, California. Though he retired in 1998, Sturges retains the title of Professor Emeritus.

As an English teacher, Sturges never quite fit the typical role. Growing up, he developed a love for words and became the editor of his junior high newspaper and high school yearbook. He then enrolled at Stanford, planning to major in journalism, but earned his degree in political science. After graduating, he held a series of jobs as a reporter and editor, though teaching wasn't on his radar.

Then, in graduate school, Sturges had the opportunity to teach a class. Scared and reluctant at first, he soon found it to his liking. He had discovered his calling. "The first semester was really tough," he said, "though I did see a way to make that better for me. It was a challenge I wanted to deal with. At that point, teaching became clear. I liked editing projects, reading papers, correcting papers with the idea of trying to help students get better at it—not as a critic but as a helper."

In other words, Sturges wasn't concerned about enforcing the standard rules of English grammar. Asked what advice he'd offer aspiring English teachers, he said: "If you're going to teach writing, don't talk a lot about how to do it; you want them to do it. You're going to encourage them and direct them, but you don't want to get in their way and you don't want to jump up and down about a misplaced modifier or double negative. Rather, keep them going, keep them writing, and keep them encouraged.

"In my writing classes, I almost always had some daily writing or ten-minute writing exercises. This was to get the words on the page. I read all that, I dated it, I kept it all, and I gave it all back to them at the end of the term. But, I rarely commented, unless there was something in it I was concerned about.

"The process and the idea of putting words on a page and getting used to that is important. The students realize they won't be pounded negatively for something they wrote. Rather, they had a reader who'd say, 'Yeah, okay. Thanks.' That's the most important thing."

His comment about not pounding students negatively awakened memories of my kindergarten teacher, Sister Marie Emelda, and the sting of her ruler against the back of my head. She clearly lacked the calmness and composure Clark Sturges displayed with his students but, to be fair, my own classroom behavior at times might have been enough to put even his equanimity to the test.

CONCLUSION

Equanimity has served me well over the years in a variety of situations. Actually, and this is a bit twisted, I make a game out of it. I find it entertaining to dial back my emotions and become eerily calm when others are "losing their cool." Much like the Rudyard Kipling poem, "If you can keep your head when all about you are losing theirs and blaming it on you..." The bottom line is that I actually do this for pragmatic reasons. If I "lose it" during a tense situation, I often have more damage control to do after the matter is resolved and tempers have cooled. So "going off on someone or some problem" actually adds to what was an already stressful day. Working through this ahead of time, helps me to keep my cool and ultimately makes me much more productive.

————— TAKEAWAYS —————

- **Control your breathing. Find a breathing routine** that works for you when you need to regain calmness and composure.

- **Be pragmatic.** Losing it never resolves the issue and typically makes it worse, so why make it harder on yourself?

- **Never raise your voice. Fight the urge** to raise your voice. Talk slowly, quietly and evenly. It's much more convincing.

- **Gain perspective.** Instead of losing your composure, ask yourself if it's really that bad. Instead of becoming heated, focus your energy on what can be done to remedy the situation. Good decisions aren't made while coming unraveled.

- **Take it outside.** Walk outside and let Mother Nature work some of her magic. Breathe in deeply, feel the sun on your face, and refocus.

- **Center yourself.** Bring your palms together, and rest your thumbs on your chest. With each exhale, focus on relaxing part of your body. Start with your forehead, and move down to your cheeks, your jaw, your neck, your shoulders, etc.

- **Be honest.** If you think you're about to lose your cool, say that you need some time to process and get back to the other person in a few hours, or a few days.

- **Let your pride kick in.** Stress has the ability to reveal character. It also has the ability to shed light on flaws. React to stress in a way you can later be proud of, as opposed to embarrassed.

- **Plan for turbulence.** Sit down and think through scenarios where things could potentially go wrong. Plan how you'd respond. Preparation will help you to stay calm when you need to most.

8

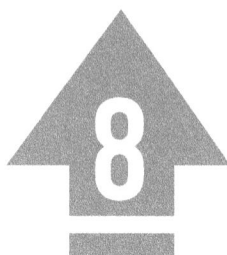

RISK TAKING: LEAVING THE NEST

Changes don't happen in the world by playing it safe;
taking risks is the way to change the world.

~ Zainab Salbi

Risk tolerance can mean many things. Some will see the title of this chapter and think about base jumping in a flying squirrel suit, or scuba diving shipwrecks. Others will interpret it as crossing an intersection on a red light or running with scissors.

Risk tolerance, at least for the purpose of this chapter, means occasionally stepping outside your comfort zone—even if your comfort zone is fairly conservative.

I have a magnetized quote on the refrigerator in my office which reads, "Life begins at the edge of your comfort zone," to remind me to continue to live a bit on the edge of my risk tolerances.

When I was in medical school, a classmate and friend of mine had just earned his private pilot certificate. Despite the fact that he was a bit of a "wild card," when he invited me to go with him on one of his first flights as a licensed pilot, I happily accepted.

My parents are not risk takers. Save for adopting me, they lived an incredibly risk free life. As I was growing up, they always warned me about the dangers of "small airplanes." I don't know why they singled out small airplanes, but for whatever reason, I was programmed at a young age to fear them. Despite, and maybe in spite of their warnings, here I was in the right seat of a small plane flying over Lake Michigan and around the suburbs of Chicago.

As is turns out (I should have already known this), my friend wasn't the cautious type and I seriously feared for my life not once, but twice while we were flying. While he was doing a "touch and go" at a small airport (land and then take off again without coming to a full stop), a car that was traveling on a road just off the end of the runway had to swerve to avoid the wheels of the plane striking its top.

This was my first—and nearly last—foray into the world of aviation, and it frankly scared the daylights out of me. Maybe my parents were right all along—small planes and private aviation were to be avoided. The problem was, despite my "near death" experience, I loved the thought of being in the air. However, to do this, I had to get over my inbred fear, which was now even more real. To make matters worse, it seemed that every time I turned on the radio I was reminded of Jim Croce, Buddy Holly, or Lynyrd Skynyrd—musicians who all died in plane crashes.

A few years later, I finally had the time and resources to start flying lessons, but first wanted to see if my fear had any basis. It did! During my first eight flights or so, my leather-jacketed, Ray-Ban wearing, Maverick "wannabe" flight instructor made me do a lot of maneuvers (stalls, steep turns, slow flight, etc.), all seemingly designed to either scare the crap out of me or make me vomit. They managed to do both.

Soon, I was running out of non-vomit stained shirts, and it was time to make a go or no-go decision. I was convinced if I could only get over my fears and nausea, I'd love being in the air. But I was still scared to death. What to do?

I approached it this way. I fast forwarded to what I'd feel like and what effect it would have on me and my future if I quit flying because of fear. I knew I'd forever regret not conquering that fear and would forever miss the freedom that comes with what pilot and poet John Magee described as having "slipped the surly bonds of earth, and danced the skies on laughter-silvered wings." That alone pushed me through my "door of fear" into the wide open landscape that comes with flying and, more importantly, with conquering fears.

When we walk to the edge of all the light we have and take the step into the darkness of the unknown, we must believe that one of two things will happen. There will be something solid for us to stand on or we will be taught to fly.

~ Patrick Overton

Most risks you evaluate will likely not include life or death—real or imagined. However, they may include loss of money, perceived self-worth, damaged ego, etc. While not life and death, these worst case outcomes are still real and may be very significant.

Identifying your fear, the basis for it, and how to mitigate the worst-case outcomes, will help you get to your door of fear. The key to get through the door, at least for me, was imagining what the future would look like if I didn't conquer my fear and what implication it would have on other parts of my life and psyche.

IN THE SHADOW OF SADDAM

I would imagine that growing up directly under the watchful eye of none other than Saddam Hussein would call for a rather high degree of risk tolerance. That's exactly what faced Zainab Salbi, whose words introduced this chapter. Somehow, I can't quite picture a situation requiring a higher level of risk tolerance than what she must have needed as a young girl.

Born in 1969, Salbi's life had begun innocently and comfortably in Baghdad, the capital of Iraq. Later, in her first book, *Between Two Worlds: Escape from Tyranny*, she would write that "growing up in Baghdad was for me probably not unlike growing up in an American suburb in the 1970s."

Then, when Salbi was eleven years old, her life immediately and dramatically changed. Saddam Hussein had recently become president of Iraq and chose Salbi's father, a well-known pilot, as his personal pilot. Hussein became a nearly constant presence, spending weekends in the home he had purchased for the family, and treating Salbi as if she were his niece. She was instructed to begin calling him "Amo," meaning "Uncle." It was, she wrote, "not out of affection but because I was afraid to say his name—Saddam Hussein—out loud. ... [He] saw no conflict between feeling fondness for people and killing them."

The family was under constant surveillance, and the tension became almost unbearable. Salbi's mother warned her: "Learn to erase your memories. He can read eyes." As Salbi grew into a young woman, her mother became increasingly alarmed, as Hussein began showing more personal interest in her daughter. So, at nineteen, Salbi was sent to the U.S. for an arranged marriage to an Iraqi stranger. Unfortunately, having finally escaped the psychological abuse from Hussein, she now found herself physically abused by her new husband and soon left him.

As it turned out, Salbi's trials had strengthened rather than weakened her. Having seen the mistreatment and suffering of women in Iraq and around the world, she decided to not only tell their story but to help them have better lives. "I couldn't find anyone doing something about the astounding injustices women were experiencing, so I decided to do something myself." And so, a self-leader was born.

Take risks. You can't fall off the bottom.

~ Barbara Proctor

"Being a leader for me," she said, "is about having the courage to speak the truth, and live the truth, despite attempts to silence our thoughts, feelings, and past experiences." In 1993, with the help of her new husband, Amjad Atallah, a Palestinian-American, she launched Women for Women International, an organization to help women in countries adversely affected by war and other conflicts.

In 2011, Salbi stepped out of an active role in the organization that, to date, has served more than 400,000 women through its team of 500 staff and trainers, helping them achieve their goals and realize their dreams. Yet, she continues to lead in other ways. For example, Salbi has written three books about her cause. Following the 2005 release of her memoir, *Between Two Worlds*, co-authored by Laurie Becklund, she wrote *The Other Side of War; Women's Stories of Survival and Hope*, which was published by *National Geographic* in 2006.

In 2013, she teamed with photographer Rennio Maifredi for a book titled *If You Knew Me You Would Care.* The pair traveled to Afghanistan, Bosnia-Herzegovina, the Democratic Republic of the Congo, and Rwanda to capture the stories of women who have survived war, violence, and poverty, and to share their hopes for the future.

In her Foreword, Academy Award-winning actress Meryl Streep wrote: "The unique approach of Zainab's book is that it has this mission: to remove the woman, the sister, the friend, from the circumstances of her victimization, and give her back due respect as someone we recognize, someone we might know."

Raised in the shadow of one of the world's most brutal dictators, Zainab Salbi risked a great deal, including life itself, to change the world. But, to make it happen, she realized someone needed to lead the way—and lead it she did.

NERVES OF STEEL

Another person who is out to change the world is a man named Elon Musk. In 1992, he arrived in the U.S at age twenty-one, ready to tackle whatever challenges and risks might stand in the way of achieving his dreams. Musk was born and raised in Pretoria, South Africa, and began showing signs of self-leadership at age ten, when he taught himself computer programming. Two years later, he sold a video game he created, earning $500. After graduating from high school, Musk relocated to Canada and then on to the U.S., where he enrolled at the University of Pennsylvania, earning bachelor's degrees in physics and economics.

In 1995, at age twenty-four, Musk moved to California, planning to pursue a doctoral degree at Stanford University. But the entrepreneurial bug that had first nibbled at him in grade school had begun chewing on him in earnest and he left Stanford almost immediately. He joined forces with his younger brother Kimbal and, financed by a $28,000 loan from their father, they launched a web software company called Zip2, marketing a city guide aimed at the newspaper industry. The company did well and, in 1999, was acquired by Compaq for more than $300 million, of which Elon Musk's share was $22 million.

His next move was to invest $10 million of those proceeds to co-found an online financial services company called X.com which, through a subsequent merger, became PayPal. In 2002, PayPal was acquired by eBay for $1.5 billion in stock. As the largest PayPal shareholder, Musk's share was $165 million.

SPACE BOUND

But his interests weren't simply to build a personal fortune. He'd long been interested in the possibility of life outside the boundaries of Planet Earth and an idea had formed in his mind. Starting in 2001, at age thirty, Musk began to set his sights on colonizing Mars. In a 2012 interview with Chris Anderson, editor-in-chief of *Wired* magazine, he explained: "I started with a crazy idea to spur the national will. I called it the Mars Oasis missions. The idea was to send a small greenhouse to the surface of Mars, packed with dehydrated nutrient gel that could be hydrated on landing. You'd wind up with this great photograph of green plants and red background—the first life on Mars, as far as we know, and the farthest that life's ever traveled."

The farthest indeed! Because both Earth and Mars have elliptical orbits around the sun (Earth being the nearer one), the distances between them vary constantly. The closest they ever get to one another is nearly 34 million miles, which happens approximately every two years. The farthest is about 250 million miles, with an average distance between them of 140 million miles.

Take risks. Ask big questions. Don't be afraid to make mistakes; if you don't make mistakes, you're not reaching far enough.

~ David Packard

Musk's idea was ridiculed by many experts, but he clearly recognized the risks involved and understood that the challenge was daunting. The costs would be astronomical, and lives would almost certainly be lost. Yet, he was determined to take the first step, which he described this way: "The revolutionary breakthrough will come with rockets that are fully and rapidly reusable. We will never conquer Mars unless we do that. It'll be too expensive. The American colonies would never have been pioneered if the ships that crossed the ocean hadn't been reusable."

In 2002, Musk used $100 million of the proceeds from the PayPal sale to launch Space Exploration Technologies, or SpaceX, where he serves as both CEO and CTO (chief technology officer). The goal—to design and build the rockets not only to reach Mars, but to also make the return trip and be used again and again. And so the race to develop recyclable rockets had begun in earnest, involving such famed entrepreneurs as Amazon's Jeff Bezos and his spaceship company, Blue Origin, and Richard Branson's Virgin Galactic.

Led by Musk, SpaceX has more than held its own. After several unsuccessful launches, the company's Falcon 9 rocket recently returned safely to Earth after launching 11 satellites into orbit.

Musk remains well aware of how much more needs to be done. "The odds of me coming into the rocket business," he says, "not knowing anything about rockets, not having ever built anything, I mean, I would have to be insane if I thought the odds were in my favor."

Don't be afraid to take a big step if one is indicated.
You can't cross a chasm in two small jumps.
~ David Lloyd George

Colonizing Mars is still far off, in years as well as in miles. In a 2011 interview, he expressed hope of landing people on the red planet within 10 to 20 years, and told one biographer that he would like to see a population of 80,000 there by 2040. How likely is it? Of course, I don't know, but I'm not inclined to bet against him.

OTHER VENTURES

As determined as he is to see life established on Mars, Musk remains actively involved in projects to benefit Planet Earth. "I'm interested," he says, "in things that change the world or that affect the future and wondrous, new technology where you see it, and you're like, 'Wow, how did that even happen? How is that possible?'"

His interest in two major projects has been driven by what he sees as the threat of global warming, and the need to combat it by developing alternatives to fossil fuels. In 2004, Musk joined the board of directors for Tesla Motors and spearheaded funding for the company, which was founded a year earlier to design and build electric cars. When the nation's financial crisis struck in 2008, he became CEO.

Tesla Motors' first all-electric vehicle was a sports car called the Roadster, introduced in 2008. Its Model S four-door sedan followed in 2012. In that same year, plans for its SUV/minivan were announced, but the car has yet to go into production. As is so often the case when sailing uncharted waters, Tesla Motors has endured its share of setbacks, some involving significant financial risks, but Musk's hand on the wheel has been steady. For the first quarter of 2013, the company enjoyed the first profit in its history. In 2015, the Model S was the world's best-selling plug-in electric vehicle.

Musk next looked to the sun as an alternative fuel source. In 2006, his cousins, Lyndon and Peter Rive, founded Solar City, for which he provided the initial funding. Today, Solar City is the nation's second largest provider of solar systems in this fast-growing field. While not actively involved in management, Musk remains the company's largest shareholder.

In 2012, *Success* magazine named Musk its "Achiever of the Year." In an article in the magazine's February 2012 issue explaining its choice, reporter Chris Raymond posed this question: "Is it courage that sets Elon Musk apart from most business leaders?" His answer: "Of course not….What makes Musk extraordinary is this: In an era when young hotshots with laptops are scrambling to launch the next Google from their dorm rooms, he chose to risk his entire net worth on three enterprises with sweeping infrastructures and steep research and development costs."

CHASING THE DEMON

Charles Elwood "Chuck" Yeager is another man who had a high level of risk tolerance, except in his case, it wasn't his fortune but his life that was frequently on the line.

Yeager was born on February 13, 1923 in the small farming community of Myra, West Virginia. As a teenager, he'd gotten his first glimpse of military life during two summers at a Citizens' Military Training Camp. He graduated from high school in 1941 and, shortly thereafter, enlisted in what was then called the U.S. Army Air Forces (USAAF). He wanted to fly, but his age and education level precluded that option and he was assigned to a base in California as an aircraft mechanic.

Following the U.S. entry into World War II, the USAAF revised its requirements and Yeager was admitted for flight training. After receiving his wings, he was trained as a fighter pilot. In November 1943, his group was shipped overseas and stationed at a Royal Air Force base in England, from which it could easily reach the enemy in Germany. On Yeager's eighth combat mission, on March 5, 1944, his plane was shot down over France. Fortunately, he was rescued by French Resistance forces, who helped him make his way to Spain. And by May 15, he had returned to his unit.

Yeager soon established himself as a highly skilled, aggressive combat pilot. In a single mission on October 12, 1944, he downed five enemy planes and, by the war's end, he had flown 61 combat missions. He elected to remain in the U.S. Air Force, which had recently been established as a separate unit from the U.S. Army. Despite not having a college education, he was assigned as a test pilot to work and fly experimental or newly designed aircraft, a move that would bring risks quite different than dodging enemy aircraft, but just as dangerous.

With the dawn of the jet era, planes were flying faster and faster, and getting closer and closer to what had become known as "the demon in the sky." That demon was the so-called "sound barrier," the point at which an aircraft would fly at the speed of sound. That speed was designated Mach 1 (760 mph at sea level and about 660 mph at the altitude Yeager flew) and, until October 14, 1947, no aircraft had ever reached it. That task was now assigned to Captain Chuck Yeager, flying a specially designed bullet-shaped plane called the Bell X-1, equipped with four rocket engines.

Early experiments had revealed that, as planes drew near the sound barrier, they'd encounter severe turbulence from the shock waves generated by such speed. Fearing, at best, some loss of control, pilots would back off, and the reputation of "the demon in the sky" kept growing. After another test pilot demanded $150,000 ($1.6 million today) to make the flight, Yeager was named to replace him. When it was announced that Yeager would be the first to confront the sound barrier, many were convinced it was a death sentence, while others reminded him to be sure to keep his life insurance in force.

What was his attitude? "You don't concentrate on risks," he said. "You concentrate on results. No risk is too great to prevent the necessary job from being done." Several weeks before the record attempt, he began a series of seven tests of his plane, each one bringing it closer and closer to Mach 1. On the sixth flight, at Mach .86 or about 567 mph he began experiencing the kind of turbulence that had scared off other pilots. On the seventh, at Mach .94, it got worse, causing him to cut his engines, jettison his fuel, and glide to a safe desert landing.

After some adjustments to the plane's tail assembly, the flight was on. Dropping from the belly of the C-47 Superfortress which had carried it aloft, Yeager took his plane to an altitude of 45,000 feet (about 8.5 miles above sea level). What happened next? Here's how he described it: "Leveling off at 42,000 feet, I had thirty percent of my fuel, so I turned on rocket chamber three and immediately reached .96 Mach. I noticed that the faster I got, the smoother the ride. Suddenly the Mach needle began to fluctuate. It went up to .965 Mach—then tipped right off the scale ... We were flying supersonic. And it was a smooth as a baby's bottom; Grandma could be sitting up there sipping lemonade."

To do anything in this world worth doing, we
must not stand back, shivering and thinking
of the cold and the danger, but jump in, and
scramble through as well as we can.

~ Sydney Smith

For Yeager, it had been like any other day at the office. He hadn't bothered to mention that, two days before the historic flight, he'd broken two ribs after being thrown from his horse. The pain would have kept him from reaching up to seal the plane's hatch. However, a buddy helped him tape a broom handle to the hatch so he could reach it, and he was up and away. Nothing was going to keep him from his date with the demon.

Yeager would continue his amazing career, and become the most famous test pilot in American history. He also remained on active duty with the U.S. Air Force until retiring in 1975. In 1953, he and his USAF team had pushed the speed record to Mach 2.44, nearly two-and-a-half times the speed of sound.

From 1955 on, he commanded various Air Force squadrons and other units. In 1966, by that time a full colonel, Yeager was given command of the Philippines-based 405th Tactical Fighter Wing, which would play a major role during the Vietnam War. Yeager himself would fly an additional 127 combat missions. In June 1969, he was promoted to brigadier general.

Following his retirement, he continued to fly for another 30 years. His last official flight for the Air Force took place on October 14, 1997, the 50th anniversary of his historic flight. Not surprisingly, he flew right through Mach 1. In a ceremony following that flight, he told the crowd: "All that I am … I owe to the Air Force." In my view, the opposite is also true.

It would take pages and pages to list the honors and awards Brigadier General Chuck Yeager has received, all of them richly deserved. Suffice it to say, he is truly an American hero.

FOLLOWING HER HEART

In our recent book, *Outliers in Law,* one of the accomplished attorneys we profiled to provide direction to students interested in a career in law was a woman named Victoria Ames. In addition to her passion for practicing a particular type of law, which is underrepresented in her industry, her risk tolerance is another characteristic that makes her an outlier.

Ames took the risk of making a career change in response to a family need. While in high school, she had developed a strong interest in pursuing a business career and spent four years in college studying for a degree in that field. Then, shortly before graduation, her oldest child, a three-year-old son, born when she was 17, was diagnosed with a life-threatening illness, for which there was no known cure. "So," she said, "I decided I needed to know more about how to help kids deal with such illnesses."

Taking the lead, Ames spent the next year studying psychology and biochemistry, finally earning her undergraduate degree in clinical psychology and human development. Finding a well-paying job in that field without a master's degree proved to be very difficult, so she went back to college for another year to earn a second degree in accounting and finance.

She began working for a large corporation, doing accounting, but soon realized something was missing. Her experience with her son's illness had touched her heart. Once again, she returned to school for further study in psychology and healthcare. After relocating from Washington, D.C. to Phoenix, she was hired by the Arizona Department of Health and Human Services, working with children and families in crisis.

Her next job was with the Make-A-Wish Foundation, where she was able to combine her skills as a business and finance professional with her passion and training in helping families and children. Three years later, she transferred to Make-A-Wish Foundation International and became its CEO. She spent the next seven years growing the organization and developing programs around the world to bring Make-A-Wish to more than 30 countries.

She loved the work but again began feeling drawn to help families and children better understand their legal rights and obligations. Another opportunity, and the risks that accompanied it, beckoned and, in 2006, she left her job and enrolled in the Sandra Day O'Connor College of Law at Arizona State University.

Every time you take a risk or move out of your comfort zone, you have a great opportunity to learn more about yourself and your capacity.

~ Jack Canfield

After graduating in 2009, she joined a large law firm doing commercial litigation, but the seed that had been planted in her heart years earlier when she learned of her son's illness continued to grow. So, in 2014, she co-founded the Artemis Law Firm in Scottsdale, Arizona. Not surprisingly, its entire practice area is dedicated to helping children and adults faced with healthcare concerns, mental health stresses, substance abuse issues, traumatic brain injuries, and other challenges.

Asked what advice she'd offer others who might wish to follow a similar path, Ames replies: "Stick with your own course because ultimately that's going to be what invigorates you and keeps you happy. And don't be afraid to fail. The greatest learning comes from the biggest mistakes."

CONCLUSION

Risk taking has marked the upward mobility of mankind. Take a moment to reflect on where the human race would be if no one ever took a risk. The first cave man or woman wouldn't have ventured outside the cave for fear of saber-toothed tigers, Magellan and Columbus wouldn't have made their discoveries, and we wouldn't travel by air, nor would we have reached the moon. In other words, taking risks and advancement go hand-in-hand and ultimately define our way of life.

Don't start with big risks, start with small calculated ones and get some "wins" and "losses" under your belt. You'll learn that the wins may not be as hard as you imagine and the losses not as tough to handle as you thought.

———————————— **TAKEAWAYS** ————————————

- **Start small** and work your way toward what you want to achieve.

- **Be daring.** When faced with the safe way or taking a chance, choose the path that causes you some anxiety, and usually has greater rewards—life is much more fun this way!

- **Assess your comfort zone.** Ask yourself if you're the type who runs toward the threat or away from it.

- **Gain confidence** by looking back on the risks you've taken. You'll see that most of these "risks" were hardly risky at all and that you'd never have learned or accomplished anything, except by taking that risk.

- **Identify** where your hesitation is coming from when faced with taking a risk. Are you afraid of failure, financial ruin, or what others may think? Ask yourself what's the worst that could possibly happen, and work back from there. Generally, the worst isn't all that bad.

- **Gain inspiration** from other great risk takers.

- **Acknowledge your fear.** By telling yourself to not be afraid, you're not allowing your body to work the way it needs to. Fear's a normal reaction; it's how you handle it that matters.

- **Fake it** 'til you make it. That'll take you a long way toward the goal.

- **Step away** from the "what if" plague. What could happen if you stopped "what if-ing"?

- **Work it.** Confidence is like a muscle; the more you use it, the stronger it gets.

CHAPTER 9

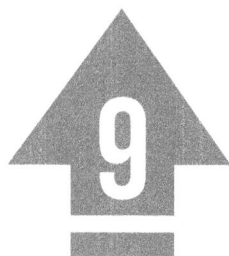

OPTIMISM: KEEP YOUR SUNNY SIDE UP

*There I was—vertically challenged, follically challenged,
a survivor of testicular cancer and a brain tumor, an arguably
washed-up former pro figure skater pushing fifty—claiming that
I was happier than I had ever been in my entire life.*

~ Scott Hamilton

Here's something I say to myself and to others very often: "If no one is dying, how bad can it be?" If you think about all the things that could potentially go wrong and none of them leads to anyone's death, then why not be optimistic?

Now, don't mistake this approach for being a "Pollyanna." Optimism is simply the best way to live. Life is so much easier when you think the best in a situation or in other people.

Optimism has served me well over the years. I suspect I was simply born this way. For as long as I can remember, I've been a "glass half full" person. Thank God, I don't have to struggle much to find the silver linings or make the best of a situation. Although my genetics helped, my experiences have regularly reinforced my unwavering optimism.

Speaking of genetics, I suspect we humans are genetically programmed to think "worst first." For example, chances are your mind goes to "negative town" when you hear, "Please come to my office, we need to talk" from your boss or teacher. Or you arrive home from work one evening and your spouse greets you with these words: "The bank called." Neither message is likely to generate a positive reaction.

So, how do you reprogram your brain to avoid wallowing in negativity when confronted with less than ideal information? First, recognize that most people's immediate default is to go to the worst case scenario. If you know you're going to react that way, start to reprogram your response early.

I start by being pragmatic. If need be, I start looking at solutions and work-arounds early. Most often, I simply conclude that the worst is generally not all that bad. Remember, if no one's dying, how bad can it be?

I also remind myself of other instances when something that seemed negative at first turned into a huge opportunity. Recognizing that perceived adversity often brings opportunity can be very reassuring.

Optimists are self-motivated by inspiring themselves to action. They believe in who they are and in what they are doing. They make mistakes and learn from them. They achieve success but don't take for granted that success will come again.

~ Ted W. Engstrom

If it isn't already innate in you, know this: optimism becomes self-perpetuating. Once you get into the habit of staying optimistic, you'll see that it often leads to success or at least provides a new perspective. That perspective helps you to see the opportunity that can result from the unintended outcome as opposed to the original goal.

A WORLD-CLASS OPTIMIST

You may not recognize the name Scott Hamilton, whose words I used to introduce this chapter, but it has long been a familiar one to me. We're in the same age range, and had both been adopted in infancy. Growing up, I played just about every sport available to kids, but whatever optimistic dreams I entertained about becoming a world-class athlete were dashed early on.

Most of my athletic career was spent on various benches, collecting splinters and only getting to play after the outcome was decided. It wasn't that I didn't care. I really cared. It was simply that, other than being tall, I possessed a scarcity of God-given physical talent.

Scott Hamilton, on the other hand, was shorter than I—much, much shorter. Given his five-foot four-inch height, plus some significant physical limitations, even modest success in sports seemed most unlikely, and any idea of him becoming a world-class athlete would have been deemed preposterous.

One of the things I like best about Hamilton's story is his attitude. Being both very short and bald—or as he put it, "vertically and follically challenged"—shows me clearly that he simply doesn't take himself too seriously. He's also a world-class optimist, in spite of the many challenges he's faced.

Optimism is a happiness magnet. If you stay positive, good things and good people will be drawn to you.

~ Mary Lou Retton

The words I quoted to begin this chapter are from the Introduction to his best-selling book, *The Great Eight: How to Be Happy Even When You Have Every Reason to Feel Miserable.* He calls it "An Optimist's Introduction."

Now you may be thinking Hamilton has lots of reasons for being an optimist. After all, he's among the greatest figure skaters in history. Between 1981 and 1984, he won four consecutive U.S. Championships and four consecutive World Championships, along with winning a gold medal in the 1984 Olympics. He then turned professional, skating for many more years. In 1990, he was inducted into the Olympic Hall of Fame and, in 1993, an Associated Press survey ranked him among the eight most popular athletes in America, far ahead of some of the biggest names in U.S. sports history, including Michael Jordan, Joe Montana, Magic Johnson and Nolan Ryan.

A UNIQUE COLLECTION

But there's another, far different part of the Scott Hamilton story. The reason he's what he humorously calls "vertically challenged" is due to a mysterious illness he contracted at age two, which caused him to stop growing. A series of tests triggered several misdiagnoses until the disease basically began to correct itself. It would be another 40 years before the real cause was discovered. It was the first of what he would later describe as his "unique collection of life-threatening diseases."

In 1997, Hamilton was diagnosed with testicular cancer, putting his skating career on hold. After a long and successful series of treatments, he was able to return to the ice. Hamilton married in 2002 and, a year later, his wife Tracie gave birth to their first son. Then, in 2004, came more bad news, when it was discovered that Hamilton had a pituitary brain tumor, which proved to be benign and was successfully treated. It turned out he'd been born with the tumor and that it had been the cause of that undiagnosed condition at age two which had blocked his growth.

Few things in the world are more powerful than a positive push. A smile. A word of optimism and hope. And you can do it when things are tough.

~ Richard M. DeVos

But there was more to come. In 2010, two years after a second son was born, that brain tumor surfaced again, which could have caused blindness, and so it was removed, seemingly without complications. Within months, however, he was back in the hospital. Doctors discovered that, during the surgery, an artery in his brain had been "nicked" and was bleeding, triggering an aneurysm, which was successfully treated.

A couple of years later, in an online video, Hamilton looked back on his life, reflecting on that "collection of life-threatening diseases." He speculated on how different his life might have been if it were not for that brain tumor, which had indirectly led him to ice skating—"Where would I be? What would I be?" he asks. He concludes with these words: "That brain tumor was the greatest gift I ever received."

The greatest gift was not any of the medals or trophies or awards or recognition he'd received in his brilliant career that topped the list. It was a brain tumor! That statement alone is indisputable evidence for me that world-class figure skater Scott Hamilton is indeed a world-class optimist.

A NEW DIRECTION

Losing one's job can also trigger negative thoughts—but it doesn't have to. For example, in 2010, Brandon Stanton lost his job as a bond trader in Chicago. That's often a traumatic experience but Stanton saw it differently. Instead of looking for another job and allowing someone else to control his future, he decided to listen to his heart and go in an entirely different direction. "I want to change the world," he said, "but I don't know how."

Life should be an adventure, to be savored from beginning to end. It is a game of constantly changing odds, constantly developing challenges, constantly opening opportunities.

~ Nido Qubein

Stanton had always liked hearing and telling stories, and he'd recently taken an interest in photography. Seeing a way to combine the two, he took the first step by moving to New York City. When asked why, Stanton replied: "The great thing about New York is that if you sit in one place long enough, the whole world comes to you."

Brimming with enthusiasm and optimism, he set a goal to photograph 10,000 people in New York City, and plot their photos on a map. He also launched a blog, which he called *Humans of New York* (HONY), but even the most optimistic dreamer couldn't have envisioned the impact it would have.

As he was taking pictures, he began interacting with his subjects and soon realized that the stories he shared alongside their portraits were powerful. Stories and portraits from the blog later turned into a book which, after only a few short weeks, became a *New York Times* bestseller. Social media helped turn Stanton into a celebrity. The HONY blog has more than sixteen million followers on Facebook and about five million on Instagram, while the book stayed on the *New York Times* bestseller list for more than six months.

Stanton's goal is to take the normal, the everyday, the mundane, and to show the beauty in that. Although the project started by taking photographs of people in New York City, Stanton later began to take trips abroad, documenting the stories and lives of everyday people living in countries we often see on the news. So far, he's traveled to nearly 20 countries, including Pakistan, Iraq, Iran, and more recently to Europe to cover the refugee crisis.

Stanton has been described as warm, empathetic, and affable. The fact that his subjects are willing to share some of their deepest fears, hopes, and struggles with a complete stranger is a testament to his trustworthiness. "What I'm always looking for," he says, "is for something the person I'm interviewing has told me that nobody else has told me. It's normally not an opinion, nor a philosophy. It's almost always a story. We all share similar philosophies and opinions on a lot of different issues, but all of our stories are our own."

In charting his own path, and using his camera lens and his storytelling, Brandon Stanton is leading the way by helping to bring this wide world we live in closer together.

Leadership comes when your hope and your
optimism are matched with a concrete vision
of the future and a way to get there.

~ Seth Godin

AN UNLIKELY OPTIMIST

As I was researching for this chapter, I wasn't surprised, given his incredible life, to read the following quote from Nelson Mandela: "I am fundamentally an optimist. Whether that comes from nature or nurture, I cannot say. Part of being optimistic is keeping one's head pointed toward the sun, one's feet moving forward. There were many dark moments when my faith in humanity was sorely tested, but I would not and could not give myself up to despair."

Like many of you, I was familiar with some of the details of Mandela's life. I knew he'd spent many years in prison and that he later became the first black president of South Africa, an amazing feat in a country with a long history of segregation. However, I had never thought of him as an optimist. As I dug a little deeper, I learned more about some of those "dark moments," which, to me, made his claim to optimism even more remarkable.

Mandela was born in 1918 in a country where apartheid—legalized racial oppression—had been practiced for decades. At the age of nine Mandela's father died and he was adopted by the local tribal chief. From an early age, Mandela became active in the anti-apartheid movement. In 1958, he and several other activists were arrested and charged with high treason against the government. His trial lasted five years and he was finally acquitted.

Around that time, the massacre of 69 unarmed black protesters spurred Mandela to more direct action against the government, eventually leading to his second arrest. In a 1964 trial, he was convicted of sabotage and conspiracy to overthrow the government, and was sentenced to life in prison. He was 46 years old.

For many years, Mandela suffered harshly at the hands of his captors. Then, in 1988, at age 70, he contracted tuberculosis. Following his recovery, he was transferred to a minimum security facility with better living conditions and, in 1990, he was freed. He'd been a prisoner for 27 years.

Mandela's release triggered a growing concern about the evils of apartheid, not only within South Africa but around the world. Taking the initiative, he played a leading role in bringing the opposing forces together. As a result of meeting regularly with President F.W. de Klerk, a historic agreement to hold a multiracial national election was reached. In 1993, the two men were jointly awarded the Nobel Peace Prize.

The historic election was held on April 27, 1994 and was easily won by Mandela's African National Congress. Shortly thereafter, the newly elected National Assembly formally elected Mandela as the nation's first black president. He agreed to serve a single term, stepping down when it ended in 1995. He was 82 years old.

Optimism is the faith that leads to achievement.
Nothing can be done without hope and confidence.

~ Helen Keller

Mandela's final 13 years were not easy ones. In 2005, his last surviving son succumbed to the HIV/Aids disease plaguing the nation. His only other son had been killed in a car crash years earlier. Mandela was hospitalized on several occasions, primarily due to lung infections related to his earlier bout with tuberculosis. On December 5, 2013, a severe respiratory infection claimed his life at age 95. Tributes immediately began coming in from around the world, mourning his death and celebrating his life, primarily for his role in ending apartheid and fostering racial reconciliation in his country.

THE TEACHER AS SELF-LEADER

I believe that, day in and day out, self-leadership is one of the most important qualities good teachers possess. One of them is a woman named Brenda Rico, whom we interviewed in our recent book, *Outliers in Education*. A veteran of nearly three decades in the classroom, she continues to bring a high level of optimism and enthusiasm to her work. Beginning as a special education teacher, Rico later moved to teaching first grade and then, about a dozen years ago, to fifth grade at Finley Farms Elementary School in Gilbert, Arizona. Asked what had led her to become a teacher, she said: "I knew I wanted to make a difference, and I thought that by being a teacher I could make a bigger difference in the world. It suited my personality type, because I like taking care of people."

With her students, one "subject" she focuses on is kindness, and leads by example, both inside and outside the classroom. "If you're constantly trying to spotlight authentic, real acts of kindness within your classroom community, the kids will want that attention so badly that they're going to continue doing it. I'll see kids being so kind to one another, and it takes my breath away. It's almost like I get to witness a miracle. To me, that's a huge accomplishment, to realize how fortunate I am. I don't know how many people in the profession get that feeling."

In 2005, in response to one little girl who was looking for ways to help other kids, she displayed her self-leadership by launching an extracurricular program called the Finley Farms Service Club. This fifth- and sixth-graders club's sole purpose is to help others in need through outreach to homeless veterans, needy children at other schools, battered women's shelters, and a variety of homeless shelters throughout the area.

The club instills the belief that even children can make positive changes in the world through their actions. Rico still operates the club, and it has become so successful that she often has to turn down students due to space restrictions.

To this day, Rico is as enthusiastic as ever about her career. "I get out of bed every morning," she says," and sometimes wonder if this is the day where I get to be swept away by the stuff that's around me, or to have a kid look at me and get what's happening at that moment. I can't even believe I get to do this for a living."

Asked if the optimistic outlook that led her to become a teacher still prevails, she replies: "I'm constantly thinking, 'I may have the kid in my room who may find the cure for cancer. I may have the first female president in my classroom.'" I, for one, wouldn't be a bit surprised.

CONCLUSION

Without optimism, there's no hope for much of anything, so, if given the choice, select positivity. Furthermore, optimism fuels growth. If you're not optimistic about an outcome, you'll never try to achieve it. At the end of the day, optimism is the root cause of the upward progression of mankind. Finally, negativity breeds more negativity—resigning yourself to a certain fate generally gets you to where you expected to be in the first place.

———— TAKEAWAYS ————

- **Count** how many times in a day you "go dark" into negativity, and work to reduce it.

- **Listen to others** who are negative and watch the body language of those with whom they're interacting. It's obvious to even a casual observer that negativity breeds negativity.

- **Get inspired;** it's amazing to watch impassioned and optimistic people infect others with their spark.

- **Pay attention** to your resting face. Check it periodically and, if your brow is furrowed, relax. Lift your eyes, and slightly smile. Practice this while refocusing, and exiting from that "dark space" of negativity.

- **Brighten up.** If you're having a terrible morning, stop at a drive-through coffee shop and treat yourself, and the person in line behind you. A simple act of kindness can easily turn your day around.

- **Rationalize** your positivity. Oftentimes, people confuse optimism with naiveté. Remind yourself that being optimistic doesn't mean you're juvenile.

- **Stop comparing** yourself to other people.

- **Focus** on the positive. You *will* see what you look for in life. Choose to see the good.

10

HUMOR: BRIGHTEN YOUR WORLD

Among other things, I think humor is a shield, a weapon, a survival kit .... Solemnity is not the answer, any more than witless and irresponsible frivolity is. I think our best chance lies in humor.

~ Ogden Nash

Among the essential qualities, the successful entrepreneur must have a sense of humor. It's what helps keep you sane. Finding humor along life's roller coaster ride will make the path much more fun and entertaining.

Problems will occur, often at the most unexpected and inopportune times. Early in my medical career as an emergency room physician, I'd started a couple of small businesses to help pay the bills; one of them was selling hot dogs. One day, a customer walked up to my hot dog stand and announced to all within earshot that I was the doctor who'd treated him in the emergency department a week earlier. This was one of those unfortunate moments. Was it embarrassing? You bet it was! But I still laugh every time I think about that story.

Humor, or at least my interpretation of it, has served me well over the years. Unfortunately, working in emergency medicine may have tainted my ability to read an audience and scale my humor accordingly.

What strikes me as funny isn't always funny to everyone or, in retrospect, even funny to me.

Recently, I was working in the emergency department during the flu season. We were really busy and our wait times were nearly an hour. Many of our patients were a bit edgy about how long it was taking. I walked into the triage room, where a young woman and her friend were waiting to be evaluated. One had a crazy red hairdo that defied gravity by literally sticking straight up. Before introducing myself, I said, "Oh, I'm so sorry, I don't think I can save you." She said, "Save me? I have a cough." "Oh," I replied, "I thought you were here for your hair—I can fix your cough. Your hair, on the other hand, is beyond help." They both started laughing, as did I.

Her friend, who was wearing a respiratory mask, had been sitting quietly off to the side awaiting her turn. I walked up and handed her my wallet. She said, "What's this for?" I responded, "Wait, I thought you were going to rob me since you had that mask on!" At that point, we all started laughing and became fast friends. The annoyance they felt for having to wait an hour was gone and I was able to sit and chat and joke with them for a bit.

If I were given the opportunity to present a gift
to the next generation, it would be the ability for
each individual to learn to laugh at himself.

~ Charles Schulz

The ability to use gentle, warm humor to diffuse a situation is a skill that can be practiced. You don't have to be a Seinfeld to use humor. I often find the best approach is to make myself the butt of the joke. This way, others generally aren't offended when I'm the punch line. Also, since I do so many ridiculous things, I'm never at a loss for material.

One form of "humor" I avoid and don't find funny is grounded in racism, sexism, bias, or hatred. Jokes like this are distasteful, and not only say something about the person saying them, but also about those who feel comfortable to freely laugh in response. Although I've said or came close to saying things in innocence that could easily be interpreted as out of line, I constantly try not to let my tongue outpace my brain. Sadly, I'm not always successful.

COMMON SENSE, DANCING

A friend and colleague of mine, a former bank president, had a large framed poster on his office wall, which read: "Business is much too important to be taken seriously." It was perhaps a reminder—to himself and to his customers—that bankers aren't always hard-hearted villains who evict little old ladies from their homes if they fall even a week behind on their mortgage payments.

At first glance, that statement may sound frivolous and contradictory but, on closer examination, it's quite true. Certainly, as an entrepreneur, business owner, or professional, the work we do should be taken seriously. However, we can be most effective when we bring a sense of humor, a cheerful spirit, and the willingness to laugh at ourselves.

The benefits of such an attitude have long been extolled by men and women in virtually every field or endeavor. The prominent 19th century psychologist and educator William James wrote: "Common sense and a sense of humor are the same thing, moving at different speeds. A sense of humor is just common sense, dancing."

Your attitude is like a box of crayons that color your world. Constantly color your picture gray, and your picture will always be bleak. Try adding some bright colors to the picture by including humor, and your picture begins to lighten up.

~ Allen Klein

Early 20th century British archeologist, soldier, and diplomat T.E. Lawrence, whose military exploits brought him fame as Lawrence of Arabia, advised: "Cling tight to your sense of humor. You will need it every day."

British-born Bertie Charles "B.C." Forbes came to the United States in 1904 and, in 1917, co-founded *Forbes* magazine. He served as editor-in-chief until his death in 1954. Today, that position, in the nearly century-old magazine, is held by his grandson Steve Forbes. Grandpa Forbes was emphatic about the importance of a good attitude for the leader. He wrote: "Cheerfulness costs nothing, yet it is beyond price. It is an asset for both business and body. The big men of today, the leaders of tomorrow, are those who can blend cheerfulness with their brains."

The incomparable Mark Twain called humor "mankind's greatest blessing." And Peggy Noonan, contemporary American author and *Wall Street Journal* columnist, described humor as "the shock absorber of life; it helps us take the blows." General Dwight D. Eisenhower, Supreme Commander of Allied Forces during World War II and subsequently the 34th President of the United States, described a sense of humor as "part of the art of leadership, of getting along with people, of getting things done."

FLYING HIGH

I can't think of a better example of a leader who has exemplified President Eisenhower's definition than Herbert David Kelleher, born in New Jersey in 1931. After graduation from college, Kelleher planned to become an attorney and earned his Juris Doctor degree from New York University School of Law. He later decided to move to Texas, where he planned to start either a law practice or a business.

The seeds of what would make Herb Kelleher famous were planted during a casual meeting with a law client and a local banker. The plan was sketched on a cocktail napkin and, in 1971, a new company named Southwest Airlines took delivery of its first plane, a Boeing 737. Today, more than 700 of that same model plane each fly an average of six flights every day! Kelleher was named president and CEO, and remained in those roles until 2001, when he turned over the responsibilities to two of his long-time team members, while remaining as chairman.

Then, Kelleher not only stepped down as chairman in 2008 but surprised many by giving up his seat on the board of directors. When asked why, he replied: "Because I didn't think it was fair [to current board members] to ... the new leadership as a totality to have me sitting there at the board table with a dyspeptic look on my face—you know, like I needed some Tums." This was a valiant demonstration of humility, with the usual flavor of humor he so regularly delivered, this time poking fun at himself.

All higher humor begins with ceasing
to take oneself seriously.

~ Herman Hesse

The story of Southwest Airlines has become the stuff of legend, shaped in large part by the personality of its long-time leader. He's been described as colorful, zany, self-deprecating, unpretentious, crazy, entertaining, and genuine. His antics have become famous. When Southwest was challenged early on for using a slogan which proved to be similar to another company's, Kelleher suggested engaging the other company's president in an arm-wrestling contest, instead of filing a lawsuit. Local media dubbed it the "Malice in Dallas," and, not surprisingly, Kelleher won.

Southwest's pilots and flight attendants are also known for various antics. When asked if the company trained them to do stand-up comedy, Kelleher explained that they're simply encouraged to be themselves. That's why, as your flight is landing during a snowstorm, you're likely to hear an intercom request for volunteers to help the crew shovel the snow from around their cars, or after a bumpy landing, a playful comment from the flight crew about the pilot's excellent flying but shaky driving abilities.

One must keep ever present a sense of humor. It depends entirely on yourself how much you see or hear or understand. But the sense of humor I have found of use in every single occasion of my life.
~ Katherine Mansfield

Kelleher was recently asked how Southwest Airlines has consistently outperformed other airlines. "The tangible things your competitors can go out and buy," he said, "but they can't buy your spirit. So it's the most powerful thing of all." He adds: "The spirit of Southwest Airlines is exuberant, it's caring, it's dedicated, it's diligent, it's fun, it's rewarding, it's a joy."

In other words, it's the mirror image of the erstwhile attorney who revolutionized the commercial airline business by the force of his cheerful personality. It's a lesson the self-leader would be wise to learn.

Attitude is the mind's paintbrush. It can color a situation gloomy or gray, or cheerful....In fact, attitudes are more important than facts.
~ Mary C. Crowley

A LIFE OF RHYME

Except for the fact that he preceded him by a century, British professor and historian Charles Kingsley might well have been describing poet Ogden Nash when he wrote: "The men who I have seen succeed best in life have always been cheerful and hopeful men, who went about their business with a smile on their faces, and took the changes and chances of this mortal life like men, facing rough and smooth alike as it comes."

Nash had a brief and rather unsuccessful "career" in the business world. He reportedly described it this way: "Came to New York to make my fortune as a bond salesman and in two years sold one bond—to my godmother." Demonstrating good self-leadership, he realized his talents lay elsewhere. "I think in terms of rhyme," he said, "and have since I was six years old."

Nash had not only a talent for rhyme, but an uncanny ability to express himself in creative, absurd, and delightful ways. Merely 68 when he died in 1971, he had written more than 500 pieces of humorous verse, often using words he'd created to complete a rhyme (Example: "If called by a panther / Don't anther.). His *New York Times* obituary reported that "his droll verse with its unconventional rhymes made him the country's best-known producer of humorous poetry."

I like nonsense, it wakes up the brain cells. Fantasy is a necessary ingredient in living. It's a way of looking at life through the wrong end of a telescope and that enables you to laugh at all of life's realities.

~ Theodor Seuss Geisel

Nash's life story was published in 2007 in a book titled *Ogden Nash: The Life and Work of America's Poet Laureate of Light Verse*, by Douglas M. Parker. Then in 2008, in a *Washington Post* review of Parker's book, Jonathan Yardley wrote this tribute to Nash: "To say that he was the best American light poet of his or any other day is true beyond argument, but it is scarcely the whole story. He was one of the best American poets of his or any other day, period, and it is a great injustice that critics customarily pigeonhole (and dismiss) him as a mere entertainer because he committed the unpardonable sin of being funny."

PICKING APPLES

Among the women featured in our recent book, *Ingredients of Outliers: Women Game Changers*, was award-winning novelist Jane Hamilton, whose writing career got its start in the unlikeliest of places—a Wisconsin apple orchard. Hamilton had recently graduated from Carleton College in Northfield, Minnesota, where she'd majored in English, and was on her way to New York to get a job. Enroute, an impulse led her to stop and visit a friend who owned an apple orchard. It was apple-picking time, and Hamilton decided to lend a hand. It would prove to be a life-changing decision.

Hamilton's mother and grandmother had both been writers, and Hamilton herself had won some prizes for poems and short stories she'd written during her school years. However, she didn't think she could make a living as a writer. "It was something I loved doing," she told us. "I loved being in that world of my own creation. It was interesting. It was rich. In a way, it was safe; I didn't have to deal with real people, which is always dangerous. I always thought I'd write, and then I'd do something else for a living, whatever that might be."

So there she was, at age 23, picking apples in Wisconsin. That was in 1980—and she's still there! "I ended up marrying my friend's cousin, who was a partner in the operation," she explained, "which turned out to be perfect because I worked very hard in the apple season and in the harvest, and in the off-season I did my writing. I had my little nook in the old farmhouse we shared with his aged aunt and other relatives."

Humor is the salt of personality. Its presence is an evidence of good nature, of an appreciation of the real values of life, and of the lack of tenseness that characterizes some people.

~ Charles Gow

It took her three years to write a short story, which she submitted to *Harper's Magazine* and, to her surprise, was accepted. That marked the beginning of what would become an award-winning career. She achieved early success in 1988 with the publication of her first novel, *The Book of Ruth*, which earned her the Great Lakes College Association New Writers Award, the Banta Award, and the Hemingway Foundation/PEN Award for First Fiction.

In addition, *The Book of Ruth* and *A Map of the World* were both selected for Oprah's Book Club, which aided in Hamilton's novels becoming worldwide best sellers. These novels were both later adapted for film. She also received *The Chicago Tribune* Heartland Prize for *The Short History of a Prince*, and her novel, *Disobedience*, was named to the School Library Journal's list of the best adult books for high school students.

In talking with Hamilton, and in reading her books, what comes through loud and clear is her warmth and sense of humor. While she is a serious writer, reviews of her novels are sprinkled with such terms as: funny and moving … charming … quirky and uproarious … engaging … exciting … lovely … witty.

It might not work for everyone, but it seems clear that life in that apple orchard, where she had originally planned to spend "a couple of weeks," has played a major role in Jane Hamilton's success.

CONCLUSION

The gentle use of warm humor helps disarm and put people at ease. Also, when encountering a tense situation, humor and a smile go a long way. I have found you can say very strongly worded messages with a warm smile and, although the person understands the words, he or she doesn't feel attacked in the delivery. Finally, laugh the hardest at yourself—before anyone else does!

──────────── **TAKEAWAYS** ────────────

- **Smile and laugh** more.

- **If you say something stupid,** laugh at yourself harder than anyone else is laughing at you.

- **Practice** using warm humor in tense situations.

- **Know your audience.** Richard Pryor wouldn't do well in a conversation with a group of conservative elderly ladies playing bridge.

- **Identify** what makes you laugh and embrace it!

- **Be careful** when it comes to sarcasm. It typically only works well if your audience knows you and your intentions well. Sarcasm plus warmth is tolerable. Sarcasm grounded in negativity is not.

- **Don't be a jerk.** Humor at the expense of someone else really isn't funny, or tasteful. Your goal is to be funny, not to be a bully.

- **Pay attention** to how your humor is received. Just because people are laughing doesn't mean you're being funny. You might just be making people uncomfortable. Know the difference between genuine amusement and awkwardness.

- **Avoid crossing the line.** Profanity, vulgarity, sexual innuendo, racial remarks and off-color humor may get some laughs from your buddies at the bar but should never be used in front of larger audiences or in your writings. You're almost certain to offend someone, so don't risk it.

A FINAL WORD

You are never given a wish without also being given the power to make it true. You may have to work for it however.
~ Richard Bach

Congratulations! You've completed the first step and, as you may know, that step is generally the hardest. Now that you're in motion, as Isaac Newton would say, you'll tend to stay in motion, and the power of *LeadershipYOU* will impact your future.

While you're already in motion, it's time to turn it up a notch; in fact, it's time to hit the afterburner. In aviation parlance, an afterburner is an extended section of a jet engine, where raw fuel is injected and ignited to increase the thrust produced by the engine. Use the knowledge you've gained as raw fuel to increase your acceleration toward your most amazing future.

In the Introduction to this book, I cited these words of speaker and author Bob Moawad: "The best day of your life is the one in which you decide your life is your own." Having decided to take control of your life, it's time to begin re-scripting your future. Whether the changes are large or small out of the gate is immaterial. The fact is that you're on your path and making lasting improvements.

The principles taught in *LeadershipYOU* are simple yet powerful. By doing my best to adhere to them, they've never steered me in the wrong direction. Keep them at the top of your mind as you travel your path toward your most amazing future. Lead your life by the system of values you hold closest; doing this will ensure that your direction will always be one in which you can take pride.

One thing to constantly remember: the fun is in the journey. You already know you'll face some setbacks. Welcome them; they're key to growth and to strengthening your resolve and perseverance. Your path won't be a straight line. Enjoy the curves and turns; they're the path to new opportunities and new perspectives. You'll meet some naysayers. Disavow them by succeeding with grace and humility. Finally, don't discount alternative paths too soon; they're often the most rewarding and enjoyable!

I'll end now with one final favorite quote from Mark Twain.

"The secret of getting ahead is getting started."

ACKNOWLEDGMENTS

I would love to name each of the individuals who has mentored me along my journey and who helped bring this book to life! Most notably my parents, Jack and Geraldine, who set the bar high and have always been there for me. To my family: René, Michael and Kaleigh, who've always grounded me with unconditional love. To my sister Barbara, who despite the miles, is a role model and lifelong ally.

This book would have stayed locked in my mind if not for the hard work of Bob Kelly, who again helped me organize my thoughts, edited, researched and drafted parts of each chapter. To my daughter Kaleigh, whose priceless perspective brought so much value to the manuscript.

The manuscript would not have come to life without the professionalism and persistent encouragement of Amanda Best, Maribeth Sublette, and Craig Kasnoff, who performed much of the heavy lifting as the draft went from ideas to words to final product.

Thanks to Vickie Mullins and Brandi Hollister of Perfect Bound Marketing + Press, the book looks and is laid out as great as it reads!

Finally, thanks to you for taking the time to read *LeadershipYOU*. I'm looking forward to our journey together!

ABOUT THE AUTHOR

Dr. John Shufeldt has nearly three decades of experience leading high performing teams as a thought leader and agent of change in the delivery of healthcare. He was an early adopter in the urgent care industry, starting one of the largest privately held urgent care groups in the U.S. Under his leadership, it grew from a single clinic to 60 clinics in six states with revenue of nearly $100 million. In 2010, he founded MeMD, a web-based virtual healthcare platform with more than 300 providers in 50 states and 3.5 million subscribers.

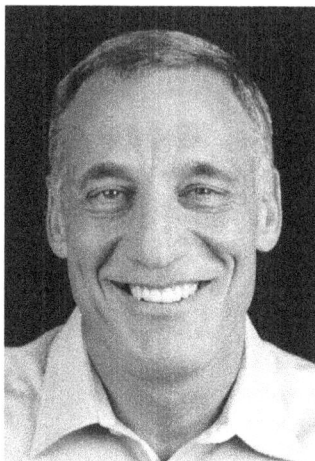

Dr. Shufeldt is a lifelong student. After completing his medical degree, he received his MBA to enrich his entrepreneurial efforts; then he completed his JD, becoming an attorney; and most recently he earned a Six Sigma Black Belt to apply lean methodology to his business practices.

He has authored and co-authored 12 books on the topics of leadership and healthcare, including *Textbook of Urgent Care Management* and *LeadershipYOU: Your Future Starts with You*. He lectures on a variety of subjects to graduate medical, business and law students and spoke at the inaugural TEDxASU.

Dr. Shufeldt practices emergency medicine and serves as the medical director for the Phoenix Police "SWAT" Special Assignment Unit. He holds an Airline Transport Pilot Rating and is type rated in a variety of multi-engine fixed and rotary wing aircraft.

Above all this, his ultimate thrill comes from mentoring. Through speaking engagements, coaching and writing, his mission is to help others exceed their own expectations, thereby realizing their dreams.

www.ingramcontent.com/pod-product-compliance
Lightning Source LLC
Chambersburg PA
CBHW060609200326
41521CB00007B/719